DOWSING
THROUGH THE
DARK

SOMETIMES, THE MORE ANSWERS SOUGHT, THE MORE QUESTIONS RAISED

LISA PERRY

Ordering Information:

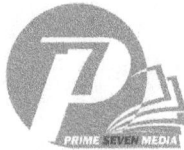

Prime Seven Media
518 Landmann St.
Tomah City, WI 54660

Printed in the United States of America

Table of Contents

PART 1 GROUND ZERO

Prologue...3

Chapter 1   Innocence, 1970...5

Chapter 2   Friends, 1988...8

Chapter 3   Love, Sweet Love 11

Chapter 4   Sounds from the Ether 21

Chapter 5   Tangled Web 27

Chapter 6   Conspiracy 31

Chapter 7   Changes...34

Chapter 8   Road Trip..38

Chapter 9   Manyip 48

Chapter 10 The Mission 55

Chapter 11 Home 67

Chapter 12 The Psychologist..70

Chapter 13 The Now..72

PART 2 AFTERMATH

Chapter 14 Prologue 77

Chapter 15 Taking the Plunge 80

Chapter 16 Twenty-First Century Disease 82

Chapter 17 My Diary 85

Chapter 18 Backyard B Lists 99

Chapter 19 Me and My Body..107

Chapter 20 Kay 139

Chapter 21 Immy 157

Chapter 22 New Directions...164

Chapter 23 How I Did It...171

Chapter 24 The Present and Bipolar Disorder 186

Epilogue...191

PART 1
Ground Zero

Prologue

Sometimes an event is like an atomic bomb that explodes the very fabric of your life. After the initial explosion, you are left wondering, shaking, dazed, and confused. Everything around you is dead. You ask yourself, *Why? Why did this happen?* Sometimes, no matter how hard you look, there is no purpose nor particular reason.

This story happened in1988. It is something that I have spent years both trying to forget and trying to understand. I still get terrifying flashbacks. The carnage has been immeasurable. I have struggled through the rubble, trying to find shreds of evidence as to what exactly caused this damage. Amongst the twisted debris I have found many possible answers, each of which has raised further questions. No answer is more plausible than the next. My memory of the event has holes in it, so forgive me if the telling is not chronological enough. I have searched in many places for the answer as to what exactly did happen during those fateful two months in summer. For instance, why were my partner Jay, and I involved? Was there a higher purpose, a mission, and if so, for whom or what? On the other hand, were we simply mad, suffering from group psychosis? If so, why didn't we exhibit any signs of this illness before?

The aftershock took me on a long, convoluted journey, one through mental illness, The UFO Club, chronic fatigue, and twenty-first century disease. It taught me how to dowse and how to listen to my intuition.

Where to start this story? Should I start from the point of impact, when it all began as an innocent ruse to alleviate boredom, or at the dentist's chair, several months after the event, when I suffered my first flashback, culminating in a nervous breakdown? I'll begin from the point of innocence and naivety …

1

$\mathcal{I}$nnocence, 1970

"**R**ight, lift your arms up," said the little girl's mother.

The young girl lifted them high and shimmied into her favourite flannelette jammies. She was tired. She'd had a big day with her mum and dad and two sisters. They were staying in a caravan in Sydney.

"Give us a kiss," said Mum.

"I don't want to go to sleep. I'm not tired," the little girl said.

What special things they had done that day! They'd gone over the big coat hanger that Daddy called the Sydney Harbour Bridge and sailed on the ferry. They'd also gone to Taronga Zoo and seen the lions and the funny chimpanzee that liked to smoke cigarette butts.

"Just hop into bed," her mother said. "You've got a big day ahead of you tomorrow. You don't want to miss out on any of that."

"No way," said the girl. "Perhaps I could have a little sleep." With that she jumped into bed, the flannelette sheets beneath her warm and cuddly to the touch. Then she snuggled up close to the hot water bottle.

"Warm enough?"

"Mmm," said the girl with a smile. "Don't forget your prayers."

"Thank you, God, for the bestest day ever. God bless Nanny and Poppy. I hope they don't miss us too much. I pray they know I love them, even if I was naughty last time I saw them. God, I promise I'll make up for it though. I'll even get them presents. God, please look after them. Amen." Immediately after this rendition, she curled up and fell asleep before her mother and father left the room.

The little girl dreamed that Poppy was standing in the doorway of the porch. The door was the old wire screen door at his house.

Poppy always growled if one of the girls banged it too loudly or didn't snib it. This time, he appeared much younger than she could remember him being. He wore the new knit cardigan that the girl's mother had given him for his birthday. It was his favourite.

She said to him, "You look really handsome, Poppy."

He responded with a nod and a smile. But as quickly as he made these gestures, he frowned and took on a look of deep sadness. He said, "Remember me, honey, by the way I rouse at you not to slam the doors and how I tell you to do your nails so that you can see the moons through them. I only do that because I love you, you know, not because I'm mean. It's so you won't get hurt."

"Of course I know that. I love you too, and those walks we have. I just get excited and forget."

"I know," Poppy said. "Don't be sad, but I've got to go away now. I won't see you for a really long time."

The girl began crying. "Why not? Don't leave! Did I do something wrong?"

"I'm going somewhere special, and you can't come along. I'm sorry," he said as he splayed out his hands and looked at them intently.

"Why can't I? I'll be good, I promise! I'll be more careful."

He looked up slowly and said to her, "It's not that. God is calling me."

"When will you be back?"

"Not until you are an old, old lady, but I'll always remember you." Pointing to his heart, he said, "I'll carry you with me inside, my sweet one. I love you. You did nothing wrong."

"Poppy, don't go." But with that her grandfather waved goodbye and walked through the open wire door, the door giving a little slap as he left.

She woke with a start shortly after that and saw in the yellow gleam of the cat's-eye clock that it was 4:00 a.m. She resettled and hugged her teddy.

Early that morning, there was an urgent rap on the caravan door, and it was followed by the sound of voices and then the little girl's mother crying. Through her mum's sobs, the girl made out that her grandpa had died at 4:00 a.m. precisely.

"Of course we'll go home immediately," said her mum.

2

Friends, 1988

"It's so good to see you, Vicki," said Amelia, looking at her friend through wire-rimmed glasses.

"You too," I said as I nodded.

I helped myself to a generous serving of red wine and then leaned back and puffed on a cigarette. I loved Amelia's company. She was fun and witty, with an acerbic tongue. We sat at a rustic wooden table on wooden chairs. I am a tall, blonde woman, whereas Amelia is short and round. A sumptuous feast of curries, pakoras, brinjal pickle, and poppadums lay before us.

Amelia asked, "How's your work going?"

"Same old, same old," I said, yawning.

"Come on, Vicki. There must be something you like about nursing."

I frowned and was silent for a moment.

"Well?" said Amelia.

"Well what?" I said and laughed. "OK! I love the oldies and the multiple sclerosis clients."

"There," said Amelia smugly. "I knew that you'd find something positive if you thought long enough."

She gulped some wine and savoured the taste of brinjal pickle on her poppadum. "Mmm. This curry is delicious."

I said, "Oh, and I forgot, it pays the bills."

Amelia looked back at me disappointedly. She was studying to be a nurse and was passionate about it.

"Tell me some stories about your theatrical days," I pleaded. "Please."

"There's nothing much to tell," said Amelia in a bored voice.

"Come on—a woman who did costumes for the Sullivans and who rubbed shoulders with famous actors and actresses?"

"It was just a job, Vicki, and it got boring waiting around, and all those shitty temperaments." Amelia's lips began to purse.

"What about that friend of yours? Mary some-kind-of-vegetable?" I said.

"Oh, you mean fruit," said Amelia. "Lime."

"That's it! Mary Lime."

"Yeah, she's fine. She's just done a play."

"That's exciting," I said.

"I really don't feel like talking about theatre now," said Amelia. She pointed her fingers down her throat as if to make herself throw up. "But I can tell you something strange that happened to her."

"OK," I said reluctantly. "What?"

"Well," said Amelia, "Mary was saying to me that she kept a journal, and she wrote in it every day. That's where she gets the ideas for her plays."

"What a great idea! I'm too slack to do it, though," I said.

"Anyway, one day she held the pen and let her mind go blank. She felt this pressure on her hand, as if an unseen hand were guiding her." Amelia paused for breath.

"And?"

"The pen started to write."

"All by its own accord?" I said.

"Yup." Amelia said and nodded.

I made the sound of the *Twilight Zone* theme. By now Amelia had my rapt attention. "What did it say?"

"That it was her spirit guide."

"Never!"

"It did. She got scared and never did it again."

"You're making this up!" I said, sucking hard on my cigarette.

"True," said Amelia.

"Cross your heart and hope to die?" I said.

"Yes."

"Maybe she imagined it," I said. "Why would a ghost want to write to someone? I think this spirit guide stuff is shit. Why pop up in a pen when they can show up in a dream, like my grandfather did once?"

"I dunno, Vicki. I'm just telling you what she told me," said Amelia. "Try it for yourself sometime."

"I might just do that if I get bored enough," I said.

"Hey, what's that I smell for dessert?" I said, changing the subject.

3

Love, Sweet Love

It was the beginning of summer and early morning. My grey-and-white cat, Ziggy, was trying to wrap herself lazily around my legs as I padded to the refrigerator and opened the door.

"Ziggy, shoo," I said somewhat shirtily. "You'll ruin my experiment." The fridge was jam-packed, and really there wasn't enough room for the experiment. "I'll drop it," I said as I tried to balance a tray of stoppered vials full of insects. It was unusual for me to see this time of day. Normally I got up at ten or eleven, not eight, but I'd stayed up all night. It was the end of term, papers were due, and I had this damn paper on the effects of climatic change on the mating habits of the *Drosophila* fly, otherwise known as the vinegar fly, to complete.

"I wish you'd stop mucking around with those bloody flies," said Georgie, who'd recently become my ex-lover. Georgie was thin, wore glasses, and was dressed in an old purple T-shirt. She pushed past me to reach the milk.

"You got in late," I said.

"Did I?" said Georgie in an absentminded manner.

I went into my room, which was my refuge. It was untidy, but amongst the jumble I could always find the bed. I flung aside clothes and pulled out the guitar. I began playing mournful love songs, allowing myself to become lost in the tragedy of it all. I had just begun reacquainting myself with my guitar. This made me take breaks from my rigid study regimen and helped me find solace in otherwise tricky situations. Dykes always seemed to try to be collected and rational, even when it came to such irrational things as lovers. I fought back the anger I felt. As a lesbian, I believed it wasn't cool to be jealous or to feel lost. I was doomed for failure on both counts. Did that mean I wasn't really a lesbian? I sometimes thought that.

Often hours went by while I played. I was oblivious to the pain in my fingers. In fact, they were so calloused that I couldn't feel much on my left fingertips. I felt lonely, despite all my friends, and terribly lost. So I poured all my emotions into the guitar.

Later that day, I handed in my last assignment for the year. I felt elated—a whole three more months until I had to go back to study! I wanted to play, to put on my party shoes and celebrate, but I felt too exhausted from the night before. So I settled for a couple of vids, a *Star Trek* and a good thriller, to keep me company. I dialled for a pizza and settled down for a night of sheer self-indulgence. I was dressed all cosily in my slippers and cotton nightshirt and was lazing on my grandmother's Victorian couch when Georgie exploded into the room with Amelia and a couple other women. The women were all happy and boisterous; they had been having a fun time at the women's pub. Some were a bit tipsy from drinking.

"G'day," they chorused.

"Hi," I replied, caught up in their infectious mood.

"Movie any good?" asked one of the women, nodding towards the TV.

"So-so. I'll flick it off if you like." With that I switched off the TV.

"Let me introduce you," said Georgie. With that she waved her hand expansively around the room. "To my right is Jay. She's from

England, on holiday, and to my left is Elke." I nodded at Elke and said hi. I'd met her before. Jay, however, made me sit up and take notice. She was a brunette with a cowlick. She kept running her hands through it because it tended to flop forwards. Jay also happened to be wearing an unwieldy pair of red plastic-framed glasses that didn't quite hide gorgeous sherry-brown eyes.

I said in a cheery voice, "Take a seat here; there's plenty of room next to me." I sat up and shuffled along the couch to make room for both Jay and Elke.

I felt myself flush as Jay sat next to me. I became aware of the flimsiness of my nightshirt as I felt the bare skin of Jay's leg brush against mine. It had been a while since I had felt this way about anyone. Last time it had been with Georgie.

Brushing my thoughts aside, I asked Jay about herself. "So, you've just finished a social science degree. How was that?"

"Hard work. But I've managed it, and now I've shouted myself a holiday," she answered.

"Wow. Lucky you! I'm broke. Did you like uni? I hated it," I said, looking into Jay's face for the first time. It was then that I felt myself fall into a space in which all I could see and sense was Jay. I became aware of Jay's bright brown eyes. *God I love those eyes! They are like liquid amber,* I thought. I suddenly became self- conscious. I had to keep myself from staring at the contours of Jay's face. I thought I'd never seen such a beautiful complexion; it was smooth and milky with a rose-petal blush. *Get a grip!* I thought. *You've just met the woman.* I wondered whether others had noticed our connection. I hastily glanced around the room, but they all seemed engrossed in their own conversations about politics and the latest law reform.

"I didn't like uni much either," said Jay. "But I want to be a social worker."

"Cool. I've always wanted to be one. I like counselling and all that stuff. I'm doing psychology, and it's tough," I said.

"Not to mention on her flatmates," chimed Georgie. "You should see the fridge. It is full of Vicki's experiment. Vinegar flies—yuk!" I shot Georgie an evil glance.

"Just joking, Vicki," said Georgie

"Sounds interesting," said Jay "Tell me about it."

"There's not much to tell," I said sheepishly. "It's just finding out whether vinegar flies do their thing in the cold or at room temperature or in the heat."

"I reckon it would be the heat," said Jay enthusiastically. "That's what I'd do if I was a vinegar fly," she said without thinking. Then once it had registered what she had said, she blushed.

"Yeah, all the hot sweatiness of bodies locking in passionate sex," quipped Georgie. Everyone seemed to look at Jay and me. Then I wondered, had they detected the connection between Jay and me, or were they simply laughing at our discomfort?

"Can we change the subject?" I said with a yawn. "These jokes are getting so ho-hum." I spent the rest of the night trying to act normal. This was hard, because the more I talked to Jay the hotter she looked.

The night sped by. I couldn't remember feeling so good for ages. Of course, the flowing of red wine kept the night going. Before long it was 2 a.m.

Georgie yawned and said in a giggly voice, "Well this little black duck's off to bed. You don't mind kipping here, do you, Jay?" Jay nodded in the affirmative. My heart skipped a beat.

"Elke, you can bunk in with me, and Jay, you can share with Vicki. That's OK, isn't it?"

"Sure," I mumbled. I looked at the ground, hoping no one would notice my flush. *What the hell am I going to do? She's gonna know I fancy her*, I worried. I steeled myself for the long night ahead. I even went and put on cotton shorty pyjamas and made sure the buttons were fastened all the way up the front.

In the bedroom, Jay noticed my guitar on the stand and picked it up. "Do you play?" she asked.

"I'm not good. But I love it. It helps me relax, you know, forget about stuff," I said.

Jay nodded and said, "I know what you mean. Are you working on a song at present?"

"Yes," I answered, "as a matter of fact I am. 'Luka.'"

"Oh, by Suzanne Vega," said Jay.

"Yes. Do you know it?"

"I do," she affirmed with a nod. "It's my favourite."

"There's this tricky bit I can't seem to get in the rhythm in," I said.

"Here, I'll show you," said Jay, leaning over me, our hands briefly touching as she did so. With that interchange, we both blushed awkwardly and pulled away.

Jay and I stayed up for hours that night, time passing by as if it were seconds. Every now and then Jay would steal a glance at me. Next time it would be me looking shyly at Jay. I noticed the smoothness of her skin and the richness of her voice as she sang. I marvelled at the deftness of Jay's fingers on the strings and gazed at her sexy hands—they were fine, delicate, and very gentle. For a moment I wondered what it would be like to be caressed by those hands. *If only*, I thought and sighed.

"What's that? said Jay

"Nothing. Except you're a great player."

"Thanks," said Jay, and our eyes met momentarily.

I broke the mood by mumbling, "I s'pose we should get some sleep. Are you tired?"

"Not really," said Jay. "But we could be keeping the others awake."

I put the guitar back in the stand. "Any preference for sides?"

"No," said Jay, and with that we both coyly hopped into bed.

Bed was unbearably hot. Both of us perched at the edges of our sides, not touching. "Well I suppose it's goodnight then," I said.

"Goodnight. I had a terrific night," said Jay.

"So did I," I replied. With that we both curled up on our respective sides. Needless to say, neither of us slept much that night. We both tossed and turned fretfully. I punched at the pillow and Jay flopped about the bed, trying to get comfortable.

I woke up early the next morning to find Jay still asleep. My heart skipped a few beats as I stole a cursory glance at her. To me, Jay looked even more attractive than she had the night before. Her hair was tousled about her, and her cheeks were rosy and smooth, like petals of a fine English rose.

I then quietly padded into the kitchen, where Georgie was hastily jamming down some cereal and gulping down the last dregs of her coffee. "Shit, I'm late," she said. "Good night last night, hey!"

"Shut up," I mumbled, determined to conceal the blush I felt rising up.

"I like Jay," said Georgie teasingly.

"Do you, now?" I said, trying to act nonchalant whilst inwardly feeling pissed off.

"Vicki likes her. Vicki likes Jay—you do like her?" taunted Georgie.

"Yeah, she seems sorta nice, if you like that sort, that is."

"Vicki's got the hots, ooh-hah. I think I'm going to ask her to stay. What do you think?" Georgie said pointedly.

"Sounds like a good idea. I'll do it. You're in a hurry," I said and then sighed. I was determined to remain cool in order to conceal the excitement I felt rising.

"Oh, that's good of you," said Georgie mockingly. "See ya, Vicki"

A little later on, everything seemed glorious to me when I brought a stash of pancakes drizzled with butter, lemon, and sugar into my bedroom. As I strode in, the sun was shining through the venetians, and I could see chunks of clear-blue sky through the slats.

"Wake up, sleepyhead," I called to Jay.

Jay stirred and wiped away the last of the sleep. "Wow, this is service! You girls are just so good," she said as I balanced a tray on her knees.

"I know, but what can you do?" I said. "I've been talking to Georgie, and we reckon it would be great if you stayed with us whilst you're in Manyip."

"You mean it?" said Jay.

"Sure do—it will be great! We can do some more jamming, go see the sights. I'm on holiday now, so we can go anywhere as long as my paid work allows it."

"You're on! I'll get my stuff from the YWCA later today."

"There's no hurry, is there?" I said. "I thought we'd have a leisurely breakfast and then go to the boat shed down at the river for a canoe and a milkshake."

"Sounds good to me," said Jay.

It was hot down by the river. The cicadas sung their love songs to us. The grasses were brown this time of year, and it was important to keep an eye out for snakes, but Jay and I didn't mind. Hell, an impending earthquake could have been forecast and we would have enjoyed ourselves, totally oblivious to the oncoming disaster. I flung out an old blanket on the grass and bought out two goblets. I popped the cork of a bottle of champagne and set about putting the camembert and paté out on plastic plates.

"What terrific service! I must come to this restaurant more often. What's the name of madam's champagne?" remarked Jay as she took a slurp.

I looked at the bottle and immediately blushed. "It's called Conquest," I said sheepishly and looked at the grass in embarrassment.

"Ooh, well, it's very nice," Jay said with a hiccup, and we both giggled. I caught her eyes then and fell into a space of absolute wonder. Her eyes. Then I did something silly and broke the moment by spilling my wine over her blouse.

"Damn! I'm sorry. I didn't mean—"

"That's OK, really. It's an old top. Let's just talk, shall we?" suggested Jay.

"You first," I said. "Let's do coming-out stories; I love them. Like, when did you first come out, and how cool were your parents about it?"

Jay said, "It was at school. The teacher."

"Not the PE teacher!" I said.

"Yes, I'm afraid it was," said Jay. "Miss … Maggie … Turner. I used to draw love hearts over my book with her initials and mine in pretty- coloured textas. I even used to ring her up and hang up when she answered. She had the most amazing voice. Sometimes I would invent aches and pains that she would have to soothe."

"Was it reciprocated?" I asked.

"I don't think so. I was so damn shy, and she was my teacher. But I knew then that I was different from the other girls."

"I know what you mean. For me it was a friend of mine when I was fourteen. Talk about beautiful! All I wanted to do was look at her, watch her play the guitar, and kiss her. None of which I got to do. I was twenty-three before I had my first lover, and that was disastrous!"

"I was twenty," confided Jay.

"Have you told your mum and dad?" I asked. That's when the tone of the day blackened. Jay became quiet and looked as if she were going to cry.

"What's the matter?" I asked.

"Both Mum and Dad are dead," she told me.

"I'm so sorry," I said. I could have kicked myself for asking such dumb questions! Me and my reporter mind, interviewing people again, always asking questions. Jay began to cry. I wrapped my arms awkwardly around her. Jay felt fragile beneath her shirt. I could feel her shaking.

From that day onwards, the pseudo- psychologist's brain in me was at work. I wanted to help Jay. I believed I understood why she suffered from depression and why she would walk for hours to get rid of her angry thoughts. I thought I knew what made this woman tick. I fell deeper and deeper in love with her. In the following weeks we both fell in love. Jay and I had so much in common. We enjoyed the same music, playing it and singing it. We would spend hours in the shed jamming, in a world of our own. On one occasion, Jay and I had been talking and I noticed that she was really angry. I suggested we play a game to help get out the aggression. I proposed boxing in which the players were only allowed to hit on the arms and the legs but not the stomach or the face.

"Yell out what makes you angry—and hit," I urged.

With that, Jay said, "For not being there." She punched, and I felt the blow.

"Great, you're getting the idea of it. It's my turn now. For study—I hate it!" Jay punched me and I flinched. We both danced around one another on my four-poster bed, toppling over and laughing as we did. This game went on for hours, and when we were done, we sprawled out on the bed, side by side.

"My knuckles hurt," said Jay.

"I ache all over,' I said. We both giggled.

"We'd better wear long sleeves for a while until the bruises fade," I suggested seriously. "It's our secret." I didn't want Georgie getting the wrong idea. Georgie hated anything to do with emotional things. She didn't understand that kind of stuff the way Jay and I did.

4

Sounds from the Ether

It had been a week full of longing and desire. Jay had gone off to Tasmania for a ten-day trek. Me? Well, I was left in Dandenong, working in the hospital for the aged. I had received several cheery postcards from Jay whilst she was away. But they had been addressed to the household; there was nothing that showed Jay's passion for me. I wanted written proof of her love, but it wasn't forthcoming, much to my chagrin. This particular day I was bored. I came home from work and picked up the guitar to take my mind off love. But the playing reminded me more of Jay. I then flicked on the TV, but it was summer viewing and the TV was full of cricket and reruns of old sitcoms, which I found as entertaining as watching paint dry. I flopped on the bed in disgust. I was lying on the bed contemplating a spider's web, when I absentmindedly picked up a notebook and pen. I let the pen rest over the clean new page, and without really thinking, I made my mind still and blank. It only took an instant, a moment of reflection to decide to let my pen go free. I felt a double image over my hand, gently sending it skimming across the page; the pen was writing automatically with me feeling a gentle pressure on my knuckles. There was no visible ghoul, no white sheets with holes in it, no howling and rattling of chains, just a gentle pressure on my hand, like that of an old woman, pressuring me to write.

I didn't have clue what was going to be written next. I felt as if I were in the head of a cranky Germanic woman, who was full of urgency and had no time for fools. "What the hell! Who are you?" I demanded. "This can't be happening."

"Molhellor Layaddey," the pen wrote.

"What are you?" I asked. This situation was unbelievable!

"Spirit guide," the pen responded. I thought I must be going mad, but I persisted out of curiosity.

"Where do you come from?"

"Glasco," she responded.

"Show me," I asked. The pen started to trace an outline on the page. I had no idea what she was drawing until the map was almost completed.

"Shit. It's the United States. How the hell? I'm hopeless at drawing maps." By now I was beginning to get a little scared. The drawing stopped, my hand was guided to a spot on the page, and the pen wrote the name Glasco next to it. Filled with dread and curiosity, I checked this in my atlas. Sure enough, in tiny print, there was a city by the name of Glasco situated in the USA where Molhellor had indicated.

"Be damned!" I said. By now my palms were sweating. I felt incredulous and curious. It was the strangest thing I had ever experienced! I briefly wondered whether I should be doing this; it was so unusual. A part of me screamed to turn back, to desist, but the psychologist/parapsychologist in me forced me onward to find out more. I found out from Molhellor that she'd died at eighty-eight and that she'd had eight children.

This communication with Molhellor felt similar to carrying on a direct line email conversation. Every now and then Molhellor would stop writing and draw the infinity symbol.

I asked, "What does this symbol mean?"

Molhellor would answer mysteriously, "There will be groups of eight meeting."

I asked, "Eight meeting for what?"

But Molhellor would only reply, "Groups of eight" and redraw the infinity symbol over and over again.

I, frustrated with this line of questioning, would ask repeatedly, "OK, what do the eight to do?"

"A mission."

"What mission?" I asked.

"There will be groups of eight. They will come."

"Whose mission?"

"God's," Molhellor replied.

"God has a mission? What is it?" I urged.

"They will come. In groups of eight," answered Molhellor.

I could feel a prickle of fear run down my back. My hands were hot and sweaty. All I could think about was telling Amelia what had happened. Amelia would know what to make of it. After all, she was the one who'd told me about this sort of stuff.

I shoved the pad under the bed and almost threw the pen away with it. Immediately I rang up Amelia, but she wasn't home or wasn't answering. I paced the room, no longer bored but frightened, with a mixture of excitement. This experience was so different from how I had imagined dealing with ghosts. *Are ghosts different than spirit guides? What is a spirit guide?* I wondered. *What does one do with a spirit guide?* Up until then my only real experience with the supernatural had been when comedians poked fun at "cosmics" who went through rebirthing and who spoke to the spirit world. I had thought new-age people were a little crazy and had vivid imaginations. I did however, believe in ghosts, because of when my grandfather had died and visited me in a dream to tell me so. But Molhellor was different. What was this mission? Finally I couldn't contain my discovery any longer. I just had to tell someone, so I decided to tell Georgie.

Georgie took the information on board gracefully. She didn't laugh at me. She was genuinely interested in my experience. "You," she said. "You need to look at it this way: you have been given an opportunity. Go for it, girl."

"That's what I thought," I said. "I've always wanted to be a parapsychologist, and now here's my chance. It's come to me."

"Well, don't get as obsessed as you did with the vinegar flies," Georgie warned. "Take your time exploring, but I don't want you driving me mad with your findings." I winced. Georgie could be cutting at times, and without meaning it she could really hurt. From then on in, I decided, I would shut Georgie out of my findings.

As the days went by, I started to regularly write to Molhellor. Hours would fly by. Unknown to me at the time, my personality was beginning to change. I started to take a different slant on life. For instance, I began to question who I was and the effect I had on life. Then there were the dreams. One night I dreamt I was on an ocean liner with crippled people. An old man who'd suffered a stroke was sitting in a wheelchair next to me. I could feel his gnarled hands and the leatheriness of his skin. He touched my hand and started crying.

"What's wrong?" I asked.

The man responded, "You help us on our journey, and you make sure we aren't afraid, even though you don't know where we're going." The next image was of the same man, standing tall and young on the other side of the gangplank. He waved and smiled, saying, "This is the other side. Thank you for being there for us." When I awoke, I wiped back a tear, for he was referring to my job as a nurse and my compassion towards the dying. *So it doesn't go unnoticed after all*, I thought.

But after the complimentary dreams came the nightmares. They were full of a man dressed in a black cowl, forever present, following me in the streets, on the tram, and even to work. The man was large and frightening; he lingered wherever I went. I think he was the devil. To avoid coming under his power, I would try not to look at his face. But try as I might, my gaze was always pulled towards him. The dream always ended with him pulling back his hood and revealing sharp, white light as bright as the sun, which burnt into my eye sockets, hurting my eyes. It was then I could feel myself being sucked into him and having difficulty pulling away. I would wake up in a cold sweat, scared and feeling alone. All these changes occurred after I'd become acquainted with Molhellor, and yet I didn't seem to connect her presence in my life to the nightmares. If I had done so, I might have rethought my decision to contact my guide.

On reflection, I realize that I never asked for concrete proof of Molhellor's validity, other than the map of America. I never, for instance, asked how my grandparents, both deceased, were doing or whether they had any messages for me. Nor did I ever set up scientific experiments to determine whether Molhellor was indeed what she claimed to be. To be fair, how would one set up an experiment to prove that one is talking to a ghost? It turned out that I didn't have much interest in contacting the dead. To be honest, the concept of the eight was wearing thin, since I wasn't finding out much more—that is, until I thought to ask whether Molhellor knew Jay's parents. This I did one night before Jay's return.

"Molhellor, do you know Jay's parents?"

"Yes," came the reply.

"Can I talk to them?"

"No." said Molhellor.

"Why not directly?"

"They are in what you might call spiritual hospital, recovering from their shock deaths."

I could feel a prickle of anticipation. If I could talk to Jay's relatives, then maybe, just maybe, Jay might be able to forgive herself for her mother's death. I knew she was on antidepressants and had anger issues related to her parents' untimely death.

"Who is their spirit guide?"

"Hector Foyley."

"Can you put me in contact with him?"

"No. Through Jay. Must show Jay. Show Jay. In a group of eight. Part of the eight." This was exciting to me, for now I had more to the puzzle of the eight—it was somehow connected to Jay's parents and to Jay. "Am I part of the eight?"

"Yes. Part of the eight. God's mission."

I had no idea about the mission or what it was, but as a child I'd been raised on a steady diet of Catholicism, on stories of Moses, of Paul/Saul, and of Mary and Joseph being talked to by the Holy Spirit and angels. I began to think that it wasn't so strange to be called— just like Saul/Paul had had been called on the road to Damascus. He would have been frightened and not known what to believe, I reasoned, so why not me? This notion went round in my head. *What if I am being called? Is it so strange to call a woman, a lesbian, an outcast?* I shook those discomforting thoughts from me. *Get a grip, Vicki,* I told myself. *There is no mission, and holier people than you would be chosen. Concentrate on how Molhellor can help Jay.* "Who's this Hector Foyley character?" I asked.

"Spirit guide, knows Jay," said Molhellor. After several hours of talking to Molhellor and some reams of paper later, I tried to settle for the night. I was excited, because Jay was coming back the next day and I could give her the news about the spirit guide. Maybe Hector could shed some light on Jay's family.

5

Tangled Web

I didn't sleep a wink all night. Jay was coming back. I felt hotly in love. It had been so long! Well, in reality it had only been ten days, but it felt like eternity. It always does when you're young and in love. I had planned the day down to a T. I would pick Jay up from the airport and whisk her back to my place, where I had a virtual restaurant waiting. I had gotten up at five and dragged the cane furniture into the bedroom. I'd placed potted plants on the table so that the room looked like some exotic garden. Then I had slowly, painstakingly, drawn menus, titling them The Parrot's Palace. I had so much to tell Jay. I had learnt a new song by Janis Ian, called "At Seventeen" and had purchased Chrissie Hynde's song "Hymn to Her." I just knew Jay would love them. Everything was perfect for her arrival. Georgie would still be in bed asleep, so I could take the opportunity to greet Jay with style without Georgie stuffing it up.

The large Boeing 747 screamed down the runway. Already heat was shimmering off the tarmac. I huffed into my hand, trying to catch a whiff of my breath. Did I smell okay? I spat on my hand and tried to pat down my flyaway hair in a last-ditch effort to look my best. I'd been up early and gone through my entire wardrobe trying to decide what to wear. Many goes and a large mountain of discarded clothes later, I decided on my new yellow shorts and purple shirt. Standing near the window, catching my reflection in the glass, I couldn't help but notice that I looked fat. *Get a grip, Vicki,* I said under my breath as I saw Jay alight from the airplane. *Not too fast, Vicki. Remember to play it cool,* I chastised privately, as I calmly strolled over towards Jay. Inwardly my legs felt like jelly, but contrary to this I was hyperactive, as my hormones were in overdrive.

I fought back a blush as I said, "Hi. Good trip?"

Jay was beaming back at me, and in a beautiful English accent she said, "It was great. It's so pretty and green."

"Not like here, is it?" I said and chuckled. We both laughed nervously and evaded one another's eyes whilst talking. Then I reached over to grab Jay's bag, and for one breath-taking moment we both fell into one another's eyes. I could see the dark irises of Jay's eyes relax and open into the soft, sherry-brown velvet.

Jay was the first to break the moment, saying, "So, what's been happening here?"

"Plenty! I've got so much to tell you," I said mysteriously.

The drive home was a blur save for the stickiness of the weather. The sky was blanketed in a sea of jacarandas. I thought I'd never seen such a glorious sight. Why, I wondered, hadn't I noticed all this beauty before?

At home, I guided Jay into the bedroom after silently mouthing to her to be quiet outside of Georgie's room.

Jay took one look at the bedroom-cum-restaurant and said, "This is terrific! You're so thoughtful."

"Here, look," I said. "I've got the tape of Chrissie Hynde singing that song about from the womb to the tomb."

"Oh, play it! It's my favourite," said Jay.

"After madam is seated in her chair," I said as I pulled out her chair.

"If madam doesn't mind, I'd rather dance," said Jay coyly. Before I knew it, we were entwined in one another's arms, kissing, dancing, and swaying to the music. I felt as if I had just melted into Jay's skin, something I had not experienced before with anyone.

After our lovemaking, Jay lay curled up in my arms. I traced my fingers over her skin and breathed in her scent.

"Jay, so much has happened. I don't know how to tell you so that it all makes sense. It doesn't really make sense to me. The strangest thing has happened. Do you believe in ghosts …?"

Jay was accepting. She didn't scoff; she simply wanted to see for herself, to contact this Molhellor Layaddey and Hector Foyley. She never questioned nor doubted the validity of what I was doing. Looking back on it now, I think it was because she was achingly desperate to reunite with her dead parents that she went along with this.

I instructed Jay by saying, "All you have to do is let your mind go blank, and let the pen carry on from there." I could feel the knot of fear tightening inside me like a noose threatening to extinguish my life's breath.

"See, like this. Are you there, Molhellor?" I said. I breathed a sigh of relief when I felt the familiar pressure of Molhellor's hand on mine. "Yes," came the reply.

"This is Jay," I said.

Jay, barely unable to conceal her eagerness, urged me to ask, "Do you know Jay's parents?"

"No. Hector Foyley. Eight will come."

"Eh? What does she mean?" said Jay.

I replied, "Hector Foyley's supposed to be your mum and dad's contact. I think he's your spirit guide.

With that Molhellor wrote, "Jay contact Hector Foyley."

"How do I do it? Let me have a go," said Jay impatiently. I handed her the pad and pen. "Here, you rest your hand on the page and let your mind go blank. You'll feel a pressure on your hand gently guiding you," I said.

"Like this?" said Jay.

The pen started slowly at first and then moved faster as it wrote in cursive, flowery writing—a completely different style than Molhellor's—the name Hector Foyley.

"Do you know Mum? Is she okay? How is she?" Jay asked urgently.

"She's fine. Loves you. Did your best. Proud of you. Sorry," came a torrent of responses.

"How's my dad?"

"Can't talk. Away," came the response.

"What do you mean, away?"

"Can't talk, away," came the repeated response.

"The eight will come. The mission," came another response from Hector.

The experience was like talking on a chat line with two disembodied voices crowding in to talk to Jay and me. One time it would be Molhellor and the next Hector.

"Hang on—one at a time," pleaded Jay.

6

Conspiracy

It was several days later, and Georgie and Amelia were out on the back veranda, sharing cool lemon drinks. The sound of the ice tinkled furiously as they became more and more earnest in their conversation. The sun was glaringly hot, and Georgie had to shield her eyes with her hand.

Georgie hoarsely whispered, "She's got a hold on Vicki. I can just tell."

"I know what you mean," said Amelia. "It's just like the sick hold Rayma had on me. I'd do anything to please her."

"Shh, keep it low. They're in the house," said Georgie. Georgie leant over and whispered in Amelia's ear. "You know she's become vegetarian. Won't eat any meat and she's lived with me for two years— me, someone who is a vegetarian! And she wouldn't have a bar of it all the time we've been together. Tolerated it she did, that's all!"

"I know what you mean. She's stopped eating pizza and won't drink alcohol; said it makes her sick," said Amelia.

"That's odd," said Georgie. "She loves a beer at the end of the day." "Another thing," Georgie went on. "They spend all day either locked in the bedroom or in the garage, jamming. Vicki's suddenly got good at music, real good. She says she can just feel the rhythm in her fingers like magic."

"And," continued Amelia, "Have you seen the reams of paper lying around the floor? She says it's from Molhellor, but it's full of symbols about God's mission. Vicki's never mentioned God before. And every time I ask about the spirit guide, she just changes the topic."

Suddenly they heard muffled voices down the corridor, and the front door slammed.

"Quick," said Amelia. "Now's our chance."

They both rushed into my room. It was full of clothes strewn over the floor and sheet music. Mounds of paper lay in a pile on the floor. Amelia tentatively picked some up and skimmed through it.

"Who the hell is Hector Foyley?"

"I dunno," said Georgie.

"This writing is all about being sorry for what Jay's done. What did she do?" wondered Amelia.

"I don't know," Georgie said again. "Here, let me look." Georgie took the paper. "What's this 'mission' stuff? Vicki hasn't said anything to me."

"I'm scared of the hold Jay has on Vicki," said Amelia, stepping back towards the bed. "What the—what's this?" she said as her foot bumped into a hardbound book. "I think it's Jay's diary. I've seen her write in it." The two women looked at each other and nodded the go- ahead to read it. After all, this was crucial to help save me, or so they thought.

"Here look at this—it says Jay thinks she's evil. The devil! That she's badly hurt her mum and it's all her fault. She sees blackness and strange things happening to her, weird things. She's seeing a shrink for feeling crazy. She has uncontrollable urges." As Amelia read on, both women felt the knot of dread tighten in their stomachs. Amelia kept skimming the diary. "It says she bonked a man. She thinks she might be pregnant!"

"She told us she was a lesbian," said Georgie. "Then why's she bothering with Vicki?"

"Heaven knows who she's been bonking in Tasmania. She's weird. I don't like what's happening," said Amelia.

Georgie said, "And have you copped the bruises on their arms and legs? Vicki said they were play-fighting. Play-fighting my foot. There's more about Hector Foyley too, how she's been waiting for someone like him to—shh! What's that?" said Georgie as they heard metal rasping in the lock.

"Quick, get out of here!" whispered Amelia, and they both fled.

7

Changes

I felt myself changing. For instance, I felt sick whenever I ate meat other than chicken and nauseous when I even thought of alcohol. This was strange, since these were indulgences I had previously enjoyed. For another thing, whenever I tried to have a cigarette, it was if my hands couldn't carry the cigarette to my mouth. I could literally feel a pressure pushing my hand away. This didn't bother me, though. I thought it to be more curious than sinister. And another thing, I was becoming artistic, drawing things and writing songs. Whatever I drew now was about the paradoxes of humanity. For example, on one half of the page would be a rocket to the moon and on the other side there would be a sketch of a starving child. The drawings were good. But I didn't normally draw, and when I had in the past, I had only been able to copy. Another thing I started to do was play rhythm on the guitar. Normally I had been shockingly bad at rhythm, but suddenly, whenever I went to strum, I would feel a force, a groove if you like, that had a mind of its own. It helped me play very innovative melodies, whereas before I hadn't been able to play anything rhythmical. The music I made was hauntingly beautiful and completely creative. I was entirely nonplussed as to where this music was coming from, but it was good, and it wasn't just me saying so.

Jay began to change as well. Our emotions, for one thing, were like a roller coaster. Serious questions about relationships and familial connections were raised. Questions that we had never thought to resolve in the past came up. These questions put our very lives under scrutiny. For instance, I'd always thought of my family as being my best friends, but I began to realize that some of this was an illusion. Yeah, sure, they wanted the best for me, but they were my parents, and I had disappointed them by being gay. In reality I was no longer their favourite golden-haired girl. I cried over that loss. Jay, too, started to get moody and depressed. She went off on long walks, unable to express her fears and anger at being left an orphan at such a young age. She'd walk for hours, or alternatively she would just sit and rock. I would accompany her on these occasions, never leaving her side. I would encourage her, soothe her, and have mock fights with her, which left large bruises. But at least it got the anger out. Whilst undergoing these emotional transformations, Jay and I would carry out written conversations with Molhellor and Hector. It was if a group of four had been formed; we corresponded daily and continuously.

I had a clear picture of Hector Foyley in my head: tall, slim, English, dark haired, with a pencil-lined moustache. He wore an early twentieth-century suit, a bowler hat, and a silver watch on a chain. His hands were long and slim, yet masculine. He felt very different from Molhellor. She, in contrast, was stout, dour of face, and Germanic. But both presences were intent on the mission. They were emphatic that the world was in danger, and somehow they believed that Jay and I would be instrumental in averting the crisis.

As if in response to this danger, both Jay and I had dreams of atomic bombs being detonated and being unable to escape the blast. Night after sweaty night we would awaken, terrified of nuclear annihilation.

We would dream images of bright blasts and blood-red skies. At those times we would cling to each other like drowning women on a lump of driftwood. We felt so powerless—and yet incensed. What could a couple of poor students do to avert such a tragedy?

Amelia and Georgie tried to warn me of Jay's power over me; they tried to tell me of Jay's mental illness, but it was hard for them to get me on my own. Whenever they did manage to, I was defensive, saying they had no right to invade Jay's privacy and that they should butt out. So the girls had to be content to watch in fear and trepidation. They were so worried that they thought of ringing my parents, but they never did because, after all, what could they prove? They even thought to hire a private detective, but for some reason that never came to pass. The only thing the girls did was to create even more distance, for it hurt too much for them to see what was going on. If I had stopped to think, I might have realized they were right. But it wasn't Jay's influence. It was Hector and Molhellor's. Nevertheless, they had reason for their concern, since both Amelia and Georgie had known me for years.

Jay and I became more and more enmeshed, however. Jay's mother appeared in the writing. The first time it happened it brought on a torrent of tears from both Jay and me. We were talking to Hector through my writing, when a different, softer, feminine personality came through.

"I'm here, love. Don't worry—it's okay."

"Is that you, Mum?" asked Jay.

"Yes, and there's nothing to worry about. You're being asked to do something important. Don't be scared, love."

"What?" said Jay. "How's Dad?"

"Your father is OK. He's in spiritual intensive care. He can't talk now. It was the way he died so traumatically and suddenly."

"Will he be away for long?" asked Jay.

"He's getting stronger, but it will be a while."

"Mum, I've got so much to tell you," said Jay.

"I know, dear. I'm so proud of you graduating and of your athletic achievements."

"Have you been with me, Mum?" said Jay.

"Yes, all the time." Both Jay and I began to cry at that.

"I've missed you," cried Jay, barely able to control the sobs.

"Me too. Jay, I can't talk long. Listen to Hector; he's got something important for you to do," said her mum.

"I'll do it, Mum—just name it," said Jay.

"The mission. Eight will come," came the masculine response of Hector Foyley.

I wasn't 100 per cent convinced that it had been Jay's mother. I also wasn't satisfied that we could do anything like a mission. The idea appealed to me, though, from my Catholic days, but realistically, how could we puny two save the world? Jay, on the other hand, was convinced and accepting of all this information that had been fed to us. She was sure she had just talked to her mother. She would have done anything for her. After all, Jay believed she had let her mum down once and she wasn't going to do it again. I, on the other hand, insisted on proof. But Jay was adamant that she knew it was her mother who had spoken to her. This resulted in many arguments, with me saying that I wouldn't cooperate with Molhellor and Hector until I knew the nature of the mission and what exactly my involvement in it was to be. A part of me, a small shred, didn't believe this whole experience was happening. It was so far out of my realm of understanding that I wanted to be damn sure Jay and I weren't going mad.

8

Road Trip

One day, after spending several hours communicating with Molhellor and Hector, I reached over and massaged Jay's forehead.

"We need a break from all this heavy stuff," I suggested. "How about we go to Manyip and see my folks? They've got this really cool townhouse, worth half a million; it's vacant at present, and they said we can use it. I've never seen it before, and I haven't been home for a year."

"I'd love to go," said Jay. "I haven't seen South Australia. Is it really that hot?"

"You'd better believe it!" I said. "We have really great beaches too! None of that pebbly stuff you're used to," I said with a laugh. "We can go home via the Great Ocean Road. I've never been that way before. and I hear it's beautiful." I took my car to be serviced; it cost me $700 but it had to be fixed, so I coughed up the money.

The day we left was hot and sunny, but luckily my air conditioner worked well. The car was jam-packed with rucksacks, guitars, sheet music, and cassettes. In a blur we waved off Amelia and Georgie and headed down the highway. Jay popped Chrissy Hynde and the Pretenders into the tape deck, and we both hummed along with the songs and looked out of the window.

"Did you bring the maps?" I asked anxiously. "I don't know how to get there without them."

"Yeah, sure; they're here somewhere," Jay said with a sigh. She'd been through the check list a hundred times. Looking out the window, she noted how brown the grass was, not like in London, and that everything looked so large, so expansive, and so dry. To me the sky outside seemed crystal blue, like the sky I remembered when I lived in Alice Springs. Those were the days when I would ride wild, bare breasted and free on my motorbike. I said impulsively, "We can stop at Port Campbell for lunch, if you like. It's a pretty seaside town, nice for romantics, I hear." Jay looked back seductively at me as we wound our way through the hills and out along the ocean. The sea to our left was turquoise blue, and the town to the right of us was quaint, with newly painted white weatherboard houses and a broad main street lined with trees.

"What do your mum and dad do?" asked Jay. "I never got around to asking that."

"They run a motel. They're managers."

"How does that feel?" asked Jay.

"I don't like it much. They're always in the public eye. Everything's so bourgeois. It's embarrassing. really. (At that stage in my life I was very political and had an open disdain for wealth. I don't now. Now I see that my ideas then were largely due to university influence and pressure from my friends to conform. Being poor, I realize now, sucks!) "Everything has to be nice and proper." When I think about it now, though, I had never really openly criticized my parents and their wealth. I'd smarted from comments made by other lesbians for having a nice car and new clothes, and now I was doing the same by putting down my parents. I shrugged. "They're nice people, but." I looked at Jay for understanding. Jay nodded in response.

"What are your sisters like?" asked Jay.

"Lillie, she's the youngest. She is great. She's with an Italian who looks like Elvis."

"The young version or the fat, flabby version?" asked Jay.

"Definitely the skinny version," I said.

"He must be quite handsome, then," said Jay.

"Oh, he is. He's OK. They haven't been married long. They live in one of Mum and Dad's flats. And Marie's married too. She lives in the country and has a couple of kids. I don't see much of her; we don't really get on."

"So your parents do have quite a bit of money?" asked Jay. It wasn't long before Jay and I were into long conversations about family and hopes and dreams, both of us laughing and talking.

"Oops," I said, "the tape's stopped. Do you want to listen to "Marlene on the Wall"? Oh, what's her name? You know," I said. "Luka "

"Oh, you mean Suzanne Vega."

"OK. Pop it in," I said. With that, we both began singing along with the tune.

Shortly afterwards, I said to Jay, "Over there looks like a nice spot. See, down this road to London Bridge and the Arch. Let's pull over there."

"Oh, do let's. Vicki, this is beautiful," said Jay, surveying the cliffs and the limestone arch that led out across the boiling turquoise water below.

Getting out of the car, "I've never been this way before," I said. I swung my arms out and twirled in the breeze. As I did, I marvelled once again at the blueness of the sky and swiped away at screaming hungry seagulls. "Let's sit here," I said as I almost fell to the ground from dizziness. The two of us sat down and opened up our picnic hamper on a red checked cloth. The hamper was crammed full of chicken legs and egg sandwiches, along with a large bowl of lettuce, cucumber, olive, and feta salad garnished with garlic and olive oil. I had packed matching plates and wine goblets and asked Jay if she would like to partake in some juice as I dished out the food with my fingers.

Jay said, "I can't remember a day more beautiful. I'm glad I met you."

"I'll drink to that," I said. "A toast to more fun-filled days."

"Hear, hear," said Jay laughingly. In the background, we heard the sound of the surf crashing below.

We devoured the meal to the very last skerrick. Driving had obviously made us hungry. When we had finished, we lay out on the cloth. Jay rested her head on my shoulder. I felt warm and tender towards her and, truth be known, perhaps a little frisky.

I stroked her forehead and said, 'We've got a long drive ahead of us, probably another eight hours. We'd better get moving.'

Jay said, "I'll get the maps, then." With that comment, I froze.

"What's wrong? Is it something I said?" asked Jay in a startled voice as she looked at my face. I felt the blood drain from my face and the most peculiar sensation, as if someone or something was trying to work my jaw and facial muscles.

"What is it, darling? Speak up—you can tell me."

I was struggling to get unknown words to my conscious mind, but finally I blurted out in a strange tone and a much deeper than usual voice, "Trust. You don't need the maps. We'll show the way."

Jay said to me, "What's wrong? You sound, different! Is that you, Mum, talking through Vicki?"

With that I managed to say in my usual voice, "There's voices wanting to talk through me, and I don't know what they're going to say next! It's not your mum."

Then I felt my mouth working furiously, and the following words came out: "Trust. We will show you we exist. We will talk through you; it is not you but our thoughts and personality coming through your vocal chords."

This sensation felt foreign, alien. I was scared! Up until then I had thought of Molhellor and Hector as similar to a dream and confined to writing. But now these words were pervading my mind without a pen! I began to cry, stating over and over that this couldn't be happening; this wasn't real!

Jay, on the other hand, was overjoyed. "Mum, I'm so glad you're here," she said.

"No, Jay, my name is Aggie, and I'm here to give you proof of our existence. We'll show you the way back to Manyip without your maps." At that comment, Jay and I both got up as if in a trance, or maybe it was just the shock of it all, and started driving towards Manyip.

For a long time afterwards, when I reflected on that day I couldn't for the life of me recall the specifics of the conversations we held with Aggie, but I remembered the gist of the conversation and the sensation. It was like travelling with three real passengers in the car- Aggie, Jay and myself. It felt that natural, and over a matter of a few hours we were chatting about the importance of my and Jay's involvement in the mission. I was still sceptical and very frightened, but Jay accepted it all as a matter of course.

The conversations went something like this: "We can't tell you the specifics of the mission until you are committed, and even then only in part, as there are enemies who would do us harm. Molhellor and Hector are involved in the mission. We asked them to recruit you," they told us.

"Who are you, then? I queried.

"All will come in time," said the voice mysteriously.

With that, I said, "I don't know which turn-off to take."

"Trust," came the voice. With that I felt a gentle, yet firm, tug on my arm. The steering wheel wobbled slightly from overcorrection, as if someone else had taken the wheel.

"How did you do that?" I said, quite taken aback.

"I told you we were real. There is no need for maps. We will show you proof." Indeed, the voice was true to its word, for when Jay and I came to Mount Gambier, a large country-sized city, they guided us through the city without a hitch.

It was ten at night when we reached Murray Bridge. The day had just flown by as if we were in another world. By this time, nothing would have surprised me, what with the steering wheel turning by itself, indicators clicking on of their own accord, and voices talking from my mouth. And yet Jay and I didn't feel a need to confer on the strange happenings. Perhaps, to put it kindly, we were both in shock and unable to comprehend what was happening. I stopped for a Coke at the Murray Bridge service station about an hour's drive from Manyip, and we both grabbed something to eat. I was anxious to get to Manyip and see my parents. Maybe they could make sense what was happening. I wanted to leave this horror ride behind me. I thought to myself, *Only an hour to go*, as we sped off in the car.

But it was then as if the entity picked up on my thoughts. The voice said, "You mustn't tell anyone. They won't believe you. They'll lock you up for being mad."

"But we have to tell someone," I pleaded as I looked over at Jay for support.

Jay just sat there with a glazed look on her face and said, "Whatever you think is best, Mum."

"It's not your bloody mum! For God's sake, Jay, she wouldn't treat you like this," I screamed. "I can't deal with this! You're not real—this isn't real. This isn't happening!" I screamed.

"Oh, we're real," said the voice in a menacing tone. With that it commanded, "Take your hands off the steering wheel."

"No, I won't. What are you going to do?" I screeched.

"Drive," said the voice. With that, Jay reached over, took my hands off the wheel, and held them down to the side. The car lurched forward, seemingly of its own volition. The indicator came on mysteriously as the car moved from one lane to the next.

All I could do was cry out, "This isn't happening! This can't be real!" The car seemed to travel like this for several minutes. Meanwhile, the voice became more insistent.

"We told you to believe, but you wouldn't. We will show you we are real."

By now tears of terror were streaming down my cheeks. "Oh God!" I cried.

The voice said, "Enough. We said we'd prove to you our existence. You will pay—you will have a crash." With that the brakes squealed on, the steering wheel whipped around, and the car sped up an embankment.

"Oh God! This is it—I'm going to die," I whimpered as I saw eucalyptus trees lit up by the headlights brush past me and heard the crash of tinkling glass. I put up a hand to protect my face. I felt the dull thud of the undercarriage scraping rock and then suddenly nothing. The car stopped on the other side of a guardrail, a few metres from an emergency phone. So all we had to do was use the phone to get help.

The disembodied voice in my head said, "Don't worry; this is staged. There will be those who will help you shortly. Stay put."

Jay looked at me and said, "Are you okay?"

"Yes, I think so," I said. We groggily got out of the car to survey the damage. On first look it didn't seem too wrecked, but when we got back into the car, we noticed that the whole undercarriage had been ripped away. The gaping hole in the floor should have meant that my legs had been torn off, but curiously I didn't sustain even a scratch.

As we sat waiting in the car for assistance, it seemed like just a moment until help came. But it was 3 a.m. For a long while afterwards I wondered where those extra five hours had gone and why all our watches and clocks read several hours fast, despite our constantly resetting them in the weeks to come.

When we got to Manyip, it was such a relief to see my mum and dad. We had decided that the voice had been right—we couldn't tell anyone about the voices. I was half hoping our experience had been nothing more than a bad dream, a figment of our imaginations.

"Have you hurt yourselves?" asked my mum. "You girls look like you're in shock."

"Here, have some brandy," proffered my dad.

"What took you so long? We expected you hours ago," said my mum.

"You know, tow trucks and stuff," I said with a shrug. The warm sensation of the brandy filled my stomach and made me a little dizzy. "If you don't mind, we ..." I looked towards Jay, "would like to go to bed. It's been a long day."

"Of course," said my parents, and they showed us to one of their motel rooms.

Normally I liked to show off the swankiness of my parents' motel rooms. My dad was a clever interior decorator, and Jay and

I had been given the executive suite, no less; it was very swish. The carpet was plush, and so were the drapes. Attractive and expensive commissioned paintings in elaborate frames hung around the room. But all I had eyes for was the bed, and I flopped down onto its soft, luxurious mattress.

"Exactly what happened tonight?" I said.

"I'm scared! They mean business," said Jay.

"We need help, but from whom?"

"That's right," said the disembodied voice, through Jay. "We told you we were real. Now do you believe us?"

The two of us nodded mutely in unison.

"What do you want us to do?" I asked.

"Go to Albany. More will come." By now we didn't have the nerve to argue. We were worried what the voice would do to us if we didn't comply. So Jay and I did the only thing we could, and that was to lie in the bed holding on to each other for dear life. Whilst lying there, I started to shake. I felt excruciating pain in my face and body. It was as if glass shards were being shoved under my skin. I began to groan with all the pain. I tried to get up to go to the toilet, but I couldn't walk; my legs were like jelly. I asked the voice what was happening to me.

"You died in the crash," it explained. "You are experiencing the pain you felt before you died and we fixed you up. We staged the accident so that we could better examine you. We are what you call extraterrestrials." I had a dim memory of a bright white light, like a spotlight, with everything drowned in eye-piercing light and me shielding my eyes but nothing else. Jay couldn't remember anything but the accident.

"What do you want of us?" said Jay. "We can't do much; we haven't got any power or influence."

"From the few comes help," said the voice. "We can all save your planet. We will show you how."

I said in a fearful voice, "I don't even know if our planet is really in danger."

The voice stated, "We will prove to you that this is indeed the case."

I said, "We need help. I want to talk to someone, perhaps my friend Kieren. She always knows what to do, and she's had experience of the supernatural." The voice went quiet then, leaving Jay and me to our thoughts and a sleepless, fear-drenched night.

9

Manyip

The Yellow Peril, as I had dubbed my station wagon, was stuffed—a complete write-off. The windscreen was smashed and the undercarriage had been ripped out.

"You girls are lucky to be alive," said my dad, shaking his head in disbelief at what he saw. "What happened?" he asked

"I dunno. I must have fallen asleep," I lied.

"Anyway, you're both safe and sound; that's the main thing," said my mum. Jay and I nodded in unison. Years later, my family would say they couldn't put their fingers on it, but on that day and the days that followed, I behaved out of character somehow. I was jittery, less confident. Me, who once rode my motorbike from Alice Springs to Manyip by myself, some eight hundred kilometres or so on a dirt road, was lacking confidence—that was unusual.

Kieren, my friend in whom we confided later that day, also noticed the change. She was worried about me, but she didn't want to betray her trust and tattle on me to my parents by saying just how crazy Jay and I sounded. After all, dobbing on each other wasn't the sort of thing good friends did. The exact specifics of Jay and I meeting with Kieren the first time, when she was bombarded with all this strange information, has been lost over time, but the gist of it went something like this.

"Kieren, am I glad to see you!" I said when I first saw her at the door. I hugged Kieren warmly and pulled back to look at her. She stood there, dark haired, prematurely greying, her freckled face wearing brown-rimmed glasses. Many people said she looked like Nana Mouskouri. "You look tired," I noted.

"It's the study," pronounced Kieren. "I've only got a week off, and then it's back to study. I'm knackered!"

I introduced Kieren to Jay. "I'm so glad to meet you at last. Vicki's told me all about you," said Kieren.

"All good, I hope," said Jay. We exchanged smiles.

"Kieren, the most amazing, scary thing has happened to us …" I then proceeded to recount our tale. When I was done, "What do you think?" I asked her. Kieren truly didn't know what to think. She had heard tales of strange energies and cars driving by themselves before. Kieren was bone-weary, but she knew it was important for her to be with me as a friend and not to judge.

"I can get the voice to talk now; if you like, she can explain things better," I said.

"Shit, what have I let myself in for?" chastised Kieren. But she listened to the voice. She admitted afterwards that she'd felt the hair on the back of her neck rising and a trickle of sweat running down her face. With each word spoken she'd dreaded what she would hear next. She said everything about the experience had been so foreign, loopy, intense, and passionate. She spoke to the voice: "You say you're on a mission to save the world. On whose authority?"

"Aggie's," said the voice.

"Who's Aggie?" asked Kieren.

"She's an extraterrestrial," I offered.

"We are to go to Albany and join up with cells of eight," Jay said. "Here, talk to her." Kieren anxiously drew on her cigarette and gulped her scotch in anticipation of what would happen next. What she saw was Jay's jaw working furiously, and then she heard a voice, similar to Jay's but deeper, coming out of her mouth. The words were slow and laboured at first, and then they gained momentum.

"My name is Aggie."

"Where do you come from?" asked Kieren.

"I come from another world. My name isn't really Aggie, but it's the closest proximity to its sound," explained Aggie.

"Where do you come from?" repeated Kieren.

"From another galaxy. We belong to what you call a federation."

"What's that?" said Kieren.

"It's a group of differing planets working together under a united force," said Aggie. Kieren looked dumbfounded. She said later that if she'd have thought about it at the time she would have asked Aggie why ghosts, spirit guides, aliens, and the mission were all intermingled like one giant sci-fi extravaganza. But she didn't, because she was so overwhelmed.

"What's this mission, then?" demanded Kieren. We were all trying to make sense of it.

"Cells of eight will form all over the world. They will stop the nuclear annihilation that is imminent in 1993," said Aggie.

"What do they have to do?" insisted Kieren.

"All will come with time. There are enemies. I cannot tell you in full."

At this moment, Jay interjected: "Kieren, haven't you always felt that you had a mission in life? Something special you were meant to do?"

"No," said Kieren.

"Well," I interrupted, "Jay and I have always known that we would have to sacrifice our lives in some way for the good of the whole. I think maybe this is it." Both Jay and I nodded. Kieren looked at us in confusion mixed with fear. She shook her head, saying, "This is too much—too much information."

"Haven't you felt powerless over the way our world is going? Felt like there is nothing you can do but watch its destruction? Well, Kieren, here's our chance to make a difference. Stand up and be counted!" I said passionately.

"No, this isn't real. Tell me more about this mission, Aggie," insisted Kieren.

"Six will come to make up the eight," said Aggie.

Kieren said, "I can't talk any more. You aren't fair. I've got to digest this; we'll have to have a break." We spent the rest of the evening recounting what had happened during the past months and hearing Kieren's tales about work and her family. All the while, Kieren's head was reeling from a case of extreme overload.

Two incidents occurred in Manyip that were instrumental in convincing Jay and me without a doubt that we had been chosen for a mission. They began a few days later when I was showing Jay the sights of Manyip.

On that particular day, the sun was shimmering off the pavement. Jay and I were dressed in shorts and summer floppy hats. We thought we'd get to the city early to evade the extremes of the midday heat. Jay was really enjoying her tour, saying that she thought Manyip to be a pretty and clean city. We were walking along the terrace under the shaded elm and jacarandas, enjoying their beauty and the cool relief, when suddenly, as we walked towards the university, our bodies seemed to fill with a rush of energy. It was if we were being driven by another force. Jay tried to walk past the university, but her feet, without her consent, took her towards the institution. The same was happening to me.

I cried out, "Stop it, Aggie!" But there came no answer, just an uncontrollable urge for both of us to walk, almost run, against our wills towards what turned out to be the library. Neither Jay nor I had been in the university grounds previously and did not have a clue where the library was before our feet dragged us to the steps. We were both frightened and annoyed at what we figured was Aggie's doing. Finally, in the silence of the library back rooms, Aggie talked to us.

"I have brought you here to show you that the world is in danger and how you are to help in averting this danger."

"What now?" said Jay, cowering.

"Run your hands over the shelf. The energy will do the rest," said Aggie. We had no choice but to comply. The energy propelled us to a specific section of the library. Our hands were automatically forced upwards and then along the outside spines of the books and journals. All in all we gathered—without even reading the titles— approximately ten books. Afterwards, Jay and I slumped down into the library chairs with the mountain of books and journals before us.

"Hey, look! All these journals and books are about nuclear proliferation and nuclear waste and laws pertaining to such," said Jay.

I was impressed. "How the hell?" Next our arms were forced to open the books and our fingers in turn were propelled down the pages. Our fingers only stopped when, according to Aggie, a specific passage was pertinent to the mission.

I said, "Jay, this is all about the mission that Aggie keeps referring to." The fact that half an hour ago we hadn't known where the library was, let alone been able to find the information without using the library's computer, convinced us that there indeed was a mission.

We were shell-shocked after that experience, so decided to go to the mall and grab an iced coffee.

"I need to sit and think. This is all too much," I said to Jay as we strode to the mall.

"I know what you mean," said Jay. "I feel the same." We entered the mall and tried to dodge the hot paving as we walked towards the fountain. That's when we heard it—the most melodic, rhythmical drumming we had ever heard. The sound drifted along the red bricks and wafted in the ether. The music had a haunting quality that filled me with utmost joy and bliss. We looked at each other.

"Isn't it beautiful?"

"What is it?"

"I've never heard that type of music before," I said. We walked towards the sound, and it wasn't long before we saw a group of neatly dressed, gentle-looking men sitting in a circle, playing drums made from kitchen implements. A crowd had gathered around them as they played, and the people looked mesmerized. In the centre of the group was a young man in his thirties, with a beard and the gentlest blue eyes. They were doing no harm, just sharing their beautiful music with the public, when up came the cops to move them on. I looked at the leader of the band then and couldn't help but notice that he had the most exquisite look of love mixed with sadness on his face. Both Jay and I couldn't help but respond to this young man's expression and be incensed by the injustice of it all. We demanded that the police let the group stay, with the result that Jay almost got arrested, and I had to fight hard not to be dragged away as well. But in the long run, the steely arm of the law prevailed, and the men were forced to move, against their will.

Later, when we were sitting down in the coffee shop, we began discussing what had happened. "The law is so punitive. The little people are forced to comply," said Jay.

"Yeah, those guys weren't doing any harm."

"That's right! The shop owners and the police have the power to enforce their will over the less powerful."

"Times haven't changed since Judeo-Christian times. Didn't that guy look like Jesus or what you'd imagine him to look like? I've often wondered whether if I met Jesus I would follow him."

"So have I," said Jay. "But look, that guy was just playing his music; he wasn't enforcing his will."

"When he looked at me for that brief moment, I knew that, had he been Jesus, I would have followed him."

"That's like now with our mission! Jesus has called, and we're answering the call."

"I think so too, Jay," I said.

"Well, maybe not Jesus, but similar, and I want to be one of those believers. Our government is corrupt, and decisions regarding our supposed welfare are taken out of our hands and put in the hands of those who are pointing nuclear weapons all over the world." With that, our fate was sealed and our pact was made. We were about to embark on a mission of the utmost importance.

10

The Mission

Jay and I looked like ungainly turtles as we scrabbled with our backpacks onto the Indian Pacific train bound for Albany.

"Whew, we just made it!" exclaimed Jay.

"I thought we were going to have an accident, the way Dad was racing to get us here on time," I said.

"Me too!" Jay nodded in agreement. We both edged our way along the crowded corridor to our compartment. We had booked a sleeper, and the tiny space was soon jam-packed with our guitars, rucksacks, an esky, and a tent. We put all our gear on the top bunk and sat on the seats underneath.

"This is exciting!" said Jay. "I've always wanted to go to Western Australia."

"Yes, Albany's a pretty town," I said.

"I wonder what the next part of the mission is," said Jay. "Aggie's pretty mysterious about it. All she said was to go to Albany."

"You know we're going to feel like gooses if nothing happens over there," I said. "Still, it will be a holiday adventure even if it doesn't."

"Do you still doubt Aggie after all this?" asked Jay.

"Not really," I said. "After what we've been through, nothing would surprise me." I gazed out the window and watched the brown landscape and barren hills slip by. "Well, whatever, we're on our way."

The trip to Albany was mainly uneventful, with few chats to Aggie. Aggie was strangely quiet throughout the journey. We didn't mind, though, and instead whiled away the time playing the guitar and singing. The days were punctuated with meal breaks in the silver-service dining carriage. It was ever so fancy, with white tablecloths and napkins and a choice of as much food as one wanted. I, who always liked to sleep in, was a bit rotten that we scored a 6:00 a.m. time slot for breakfast. But caught between the prospects of having breakfast and sleeping in, having breakfast won hands down.

The night before we reached Albany, I had another one of my nightmares. It was of a man dressed in a black cowl. He was standing at the edge of the train bunk, with his robes flapping. He was much closer to me than he'd ever been before. His fingers looked like gnarled roots as he pushed back his hood to reveal a blinding light. I sweated profusely as I tried to shield my eyes. I struggled to get up, to do anything to escape him. It was as if he wanted something. I thought it was my soul. He reached towards me with his gnarly hand, almost clasping my T-shirt. I couldn't move but only lay there. Luckily, I suddenly woke up when the train slowed around a corner with a squeal of its brakes.

Afterwards I stayed awake, staring sightlessly into the dark until daybreak. All that morning, and when Jay eventually woke, I was quiet and withdrawn, inwardly wondering what we had gotten ourselves into. In order to allay my fears, I looked for omens that everything would be all right. In fact, Jay and I felt it to be a good sign that we arrived in Albany on Good Friday, which made us feel that at least in some way we were following Christ's journey. As a result, we both felt our spirits lift. Another omen was the number of the caravan park we chose to stay at. We took this as a symbol: it was at number 38 on the street. The three represented the holy trinity with

Christ, and the eight represented the groups of eight that would form together to save the world. Both of us excitedly discussed this notion as we entered the caravan park.

It was only when we were inside the park that we noticed our surroundings. We were situated on the banks of a river that was lined with tall eucalypts. The tent site was mown grass and well cared for. Had we thought as we staggered with our luggage to our prospective tent site that day about what we would do for money, jobs, and transport, we would have panicked. But instead, we were so intent with the mission that we just set up camp and literally waited for the next set of instructions from Aggie.

These instructions were slow in coming. Instead Aggie filled in our time with explanations of her world. Aggie spoke these words through me. The conversation came in the form of a three-person dialogue, with me being totally unaware of what Aggie was going to say until the words were uttered from my mouth.

"We look like your reptiles, but we're bipedal and approximately your height."

"Is your skin scaly?" asked Jay.

Laughing, Aggie told us it was like that of a lizard.

"What's your planet like?" I said.

"It's dry, with large white rock formations. We have very little water and two moons."

"Two moons!" said Jay.

"Yes, like silver wedges hanging in the sky. We live underground, you know, in domes shaped out of mud and a rock-like substance, which is highly sophisticated. The sky at night is a deep indigo, and when I go flying my ship, I can see large canyons that wind on for miles."

"Do you wear clothes?" asked Jay coyly.

"Yes, a sort of silver uniform. We wear a *shukta* around our foreheads to protect our third eyes. It's a stone like a ruby; its energy is thought to protect and heal. I am a healer. We use minerals and the vibrations from them to heal."

"So there is some truth to energy healing with stones?" I asked.

"There certainly is, but ours is connected to equipment that enhances these qualities."

"Wow!" said Jay.

"Do you have males and females?" asked Jay shyly.

"No, we are what you call both in the one body."

"How do you reproduce, then?" I said with a tone of incredulousness.

"That would be telling," Aggie said with a laugh. "We have a special ritual called *deenaht* that occurs once every six months, whereby we can choose to carry a child if we wish." I wanted to hear more, but my butt was numb, it was unbearably hot in the tent, and it smelt of sweat and mown grass. I jumped up quickly and impatiently unzipped the tent, trying to swish in some fresh, cool air.

"There, that's better. Go on," I said.

"Are you monogamous?" asked Jay, barely able to conceal her interest.

"No. We form clans connected by mutual affection, respect, and dignity. We do not believe monogamy is just."

Jay looked at me and nodded. "It can be lonely when you're the one on the outside."

Fascinated, I asked, "How is your government run?"

"We have a federation of planets; we do not come from one planet but many. We were the first to inhabit your planet."

"No!" we chorused.

"About three and a half million years ago."

"What happened? Why don't we look like you?" asked Jay.

"A disease killed most of the settlers before we could evacuate this planet. We don't have a cure for the disease. Our federation has evolved so that it oversees planets now, and we are not to become directly involved with planets' politics. That is why we abduct people, so that individuals can work towards the survival of the planet."

"If you're talking to us like this, why do you need to abduct?"

"Because we're often not heard this way, and if we are we are, we're not believed. They see it as madness. Just like you do."

"You've got a point there," we chimed.

"If you showed up in person, we would believe," I said.

"I know, but we cannot risk ourselves to the spores of the disease."

I suggested, "Why not speak to our governments directly? Point out the danger we are in. We're starving for outside influence and guidance."

"You could broadcast yourself on TV."

"The government would only see it as a hoax," said Aggie sadly.

"But you could make them believe. Show your spaceship," said Jay. "It's as if Earth is this one big, lonely child looking for a mentor."

"You mean like the Vulcans in *Star Trek* were to Earth?" I said.

"Yeah, sort of," mumbled Jay, shifting uncomfortably in her cramped position.

"We tried that. But your governments exploited our tools and used them as weapons. Like the stealth bomber. To us, stealth bombers were recognizance ships used to avoid clashes, not to fight wars with. Not to mention some of your laser technology. No, it is better that we do it this way, with the people not creating a stir."

"Ooh, ooh, this is so interesting, but I have to do a wee," said Jay.

"And my foot's gone to sleep," I said, stamping my foot on the ground and trying desperately to get the circulation back in my cramped limbs.

Jay almost crashed past me in her desperation to go to the loo.

"So, what do you do for fun?" I said, and then, "This is crazy! I'm talking to myself and I'm answering back." I shook my head, still having some lingering doubts regarding the previous conversation. With Jay present I knew I wasn't crazy, but when she was gone, my doubts were raised. I shook my head, terminating the conversation with Aggie, and pushed my head out into the bright sunshine outside the tent flap, gulping in the fresh air.

About twenty minutes later Jay came back to the tent flushed and excited. She'd told me she'd met some really amazing people who were camping only a few tent sites away. She'd met this woman called Kay in the loo and had started chatting to her about the weather and asked her what sort of day she'd had. That, Jay exclaimed, is what made her interesting—she'd been trying to organize a pyramid healing centre throughout Australia, which involved meditation and healing energy that incorporated using stones. Jay got all excited and asked me whether we dared talk to them about our experiences.

"It's worth further investigation, at least," I said logically. Inwardly I wanted—needed—to confide in someone neutral, someone who wouldn't judge but would listen and maybe even offer some advice. I was scared of what was happening to us both. To me it seemed that Jay accepted it all in her stride, while I, on the other hand, was having difficulty with it all. If only there were someone else … But outwardly I shrugged, saying, "I'd like to find out more about them. They could be kooks, for all we know!"

We met up with Kay and her husband, Kerry, shortly afterwards. They were sitting in striped deckchairs in the shade next to their caravan. It was a quaint old wooden box on wheels, freshly painted. It was hitched to a closed trailer, which was full of books.

The first thing I noticed about Kerry was his eyes. They were blue and intense, as if they could see right into the very core of my being. They were the sort of eyes that you couldn't lie to, eyes that only told the truth.

Seeing us gaze at the trailer, Kerry waved expansively with a spidery arm and said, "I love books."

"Gee. You must to carry a whole trailer load," said Jay.

"We've got so many books because we're going to set up our healing business," said Kerry.

"Take a seat," proffered Kay. "We like good company." Jay liked the sound of Kay's voice; it jingled in a singsong sort of way. Jay saw in Kay's round face kindness and openness, so much so that she wanted tell our story then and there. She looked at me, but I shook my head in disagreement.

So instead Jay said, "We're here on a sort of working holiday. Vicki's a nurse, and I'm looking for casual work." I nodded in agreement.

"I'm waiting to get clear swabs, so's I can work in Albany hospitals, but it's taking time, it's hot, and we're running low on money."

"That's hard," said Kay empathically.

"Cigarette?" offered Kerry.

"No, thanks; I'm trying to give up," I said.

"Kerry consciously smokes," said Kay.

"What's that mean?" I asked.

"It means that I cut down, for a start, and I stop blaming myself for enjoying the occasional cigarette."

"In that case, can I try?" Kerry gave me a cigarette, which I hurriedly lit and dragged heavily on through the filter. I felt the smoke fill my lungs and serenity extend throughout my entire body. *There, that's better. I consciously accept this cigarette.* "Hey, it works!"

"I told you so," said Kay.

"Exactly. If you smoke consciously, you want less and enjoy more."

Jay said impatiently, "Should we tell them?"

"Sh," I said.

"What's that? If we can help in any way," said Kay sympathetically.

"But you don't know us from a bar of soap," I said.

"Let us be the judge of that. I'm a good arbiter of character," said Kerry.

Jay spoke passionately: "If we don't tell someone, we'll go mad!"

I mumbled, "You're right. It started like this …" A knot of dread tightened in my stomach as I began.

At the end of the tale, Kerry's earnest eyes revealed belief. He said, "My mission is to set up pyramid centres around Australia. Perhaps, as both Kay and I are doing the Course in Miracles, we were destined to meet you. We've met others who have had alien children. Do the aliens look like this?" He showed us a book with a drawing of a figure exactly the same as had been described by Aggie—right up to the shuktah (the stone) worn over the third eye.

"Yes, but how?" said Jay and I in unison.

"We've known about this race for a long time. They are connected to the beings from Lemuria."

"But that's a myth. It's a mythical place in America," said Jay knowingly.

"Is it? How can you explain that your alien looks like this one, then?

"I can't," admitted Jay.

"Neither can I," said Kerry. "Can we talk with the voice?"

"I think so," I said, though I was somewhat dubious. "I feel like she wants to talk to you, because my mouth feels like it wants to speak, but I don't know what it will say."

"Aggie!" I called.

Aggie spoke in her familiar tone: "Greetings. At last we meet. I have guided these two to you. You are to be involved on a mission of the gravest importance. The world is in danger."

"What do you want us to do?" asked Kerry.

"You will eventually form a group of eight. Now you are six, counting myself and Hector. You will be asked to wait for instructions."

"Tell us about yourselves," asked Kerry

"We are a federation wanting to save your world. You are being judged on the importance of your planet. We have come to intervene. We are to decide whether the Earth should be destroyed or not.

"When they come, you must speak your truth."

"Who's *they*?" asked Kerry.

"You who have been chosen."

"But what for? And how?" asked Kay.

"They will come. When the time is right. Meanwhile, you must prepare your vessels."

"Vessels? What are our vessels?" I asked.

"Your body, mind, and spirit. Kerry and Kay must do this."

"You mean rebirthing?" said Kerry excitedly.

"Yes. Exactly."

To me, rebirthing was the butt of feminist jokes. I remembered a skit wherein a woman wore a bathing cap and snorkel for her rebirthing. I had shrieked with laughter then at the absurdity of someone plunging to the depths of her own soul.

I asked now, "What's rebirthing?"

Kerry answered, "It's like hypnotherapy. We regress you through the traumatic blocks in your life and other lifetimes so that they don't stop your growth in this lifetime."

"Why do we have to do that? Aren't we all right?" I said.

Aggie answered, "To be the best at this mission, it is important that you do this."

Jay said, "Come on, Vicki; this is important."

"I'm not happy about it, but I'll give it a go. There's none of that cosmic stuff, is there?" I said.

"It's relatively straightforward," said Kay. "We've done it many times before."

With that, I reluctantly agreed. "I think we should call it quits for the day. My brain is aching from all this information." Then we settled down to mandarin and ginger herbal tea drinks.

Later that day, as the midday sun was burning brightly in the sky, Jay and I had left Kerry and Kay to beat the heat. We stripped off to bare essentials and slopped sunscreen over our bodies. The sweat trickled down our noses, and our skin became greasy from oil. We plunged our feet through the icy skin of the river, and clouds of oil formed a scum on the surface of the water.

"Ooh, that's better," I said. We both hooked up our pants and ventured further in. My legs tingled with the coolness of it; it ran right up to the pit of my stomach.

"I dunno. What do you think of Kay and Kerry?" I asked.

"They seem nice," responded Jay.

"I think they seem a bit cosmic."

"So do we! Our car driving by itself. Missions from aliens."

"I s'pose."

"They seem genuine."

"They do," I said with a nod.

"It's so good to unload some of this stuff. I thought I was going to go mad," said Jay. I nodded again in agreement.

"We need to find somewhere else to live. It's too hot here."

"You're not kidding," I said.

"I've found somewhere we can stay through Lesbian Network. Let's try it out, shall we?"

"Anywhere's better than being in this heat."

The Lesbian Network turned out to be fruitful for us. We found a flat in Albany, near the gardens. It was free accommodation, because the woman who owned it was away for several months and she needed the flat to be looked after. It was another sign for us that everything was meant to be.

"Look!" I pointed out to Jay. "Its number is 38." I could barely contain my amazement. I had to admit these signs seemed very encouraging. I looked at the grey stone flat. Not bad. I ran my hand along a rusted handrail. It felt burning hot as I walked up the flight of stairs to a quaint entrance. As I did so, I huffed slightly from the heat.

To the west was a park full of sinewy, sensuous eucalypts. The dying sun shot golden fingers of sunlight on the tips of the trees. I held my breath as I watched the crimson light dropping slowly in the sky.

"Nice to meet you at last," I said to Deidre, the women from Lesbian Network. Deidre's grip was strong and firm. I noticed that her hands were the hands of someone used to the earth, for they were calloused, with ingrained dirt.

"What a lovely feeling flat," said Jay. I breathed deeply and smelt the faint odour of sandalwood in the air. It reminded me of happy days back in Dandenong, with Josie and Georgie, and of long talks, bacon and eggs, and safety. I ran my hand over an exquisite piece of driftwood.

"I love this sort of stuff. Ooh, and she's got a baobab nut! I've always wanted to see what they're like inside. I picked up the nut, felt the firm fuzzy covering, and rolled it around in my hands before placing it gently to my cheek. "It feels so nice."

"Yes, Danny loves nature. She is a painter, as you can tell." Deidre waved expansively around the room.

"They're gorgeous," I said. "Did she paint all of them?"

"Mostly." The paintings were pen and wash and were of natural objects in nature. I became aware of Deidre's obvious pride in the paintings and asked, "Are you and Danny lovers?" I detected a blush.

"No, no. We're just good friends."

I decided not to push the topic but instead said, "May I look at the bedroom?"

"It's to the right.

The first thing I noticed was how airy the room was. It had a large window overlooking the city skyline. The blueness of the walls gave the room a fresh feel. A double mattress was on the floor, and above the bed hung a beautiful maroon-and-blue cardboard star that wafted in the gentle breeze blowing through the open window.

"I'm impressed," I said. "This is great."

"It *is* great," said Jay, plopping down on the mattress. "And the bed's comfy too." "When can we move in?" I asked.

"Straight away, if you like."

"Magic," said Jay and I in unison.

11

Home

During the next few weeks, Kerry and Kay came over to our flat to do our rebirthing. Forgive me if my memory fails me of exactly what happened during those weeks. I have vivid flashes intermingled with feelings of fear of that time. Needless to say, the rebirthing was too much for my mind to deal with. That, coupled with the experiences we'd had previously, culminated in a meltdown.

Two things I do remember. First, in my mind's eye, I was confronted by two beings who were trying to determine whether humanity should be annihilated or not. It was then that we met as a circle of eight, comprising Hector, Aggie, Kerry, Kay, Jay myself, and the two prosecuting beings. The room became like a courtroom, and Jay and I were the defendants. We won for Earth after a lengthy debate. The verdict was given that in 1993 aliens would help avert Earth's nuclear destruction.

The other experience I remember was that I became possessed by the devil. It was terrifying! I felt that my soul was being sucked out of my very being. Kerry, Kay, Jay, and I ended up at a church, begging the local chaplain to do an exorcism on me, which he did. I immediately felt better, for I could feel the dark energy leave me, but I remained terrified for a long time after that ordeal.

Immediately after the exorcism, we were sitting in a circle in our flat, discussing what we should do next, when the phone rang. It was my parents. When I heard my mother's voice, I sobbed. "Do you love me, Mum and Dad? "Everything's gone wrong here. We're in terrible trouble!"

"What's wrong? I'll fly up and get you," said my dad.

"No. No, I just want to come home."

At that, Kerry took the phone and explained that I'd had some sort of breakdown and that it was best I went home to them. It was the first time I had heard of it, but I was so eager to go home, I just complied. I didn't want to be on a mission any longer; I wanted to be ordinary Vicki Frances.

I was bundled up in a hurry. Jay remained behind. She looked as though she had lost it, for she was quietly humming, with a faraway look in her eyes, whilst holding a metal pyramid over her head. To tell the truth, I didn't give much thought to anyone while I was being packed up. All I wanted was to go home.

I remember the flight in and overlooking the familiar sights of Manyip. The sky was a sparkling blue, and the ocean danced up to greet me as the plane did the final circle towards the brown grassiness of the airstrip. It was magic. I was wondering, had my experiences been a terrible dream? But I lost that thought when I saw the concerned faces of Mum and Dad greeting me.

Though I might try, how could I adequately explain what I had experienced? Dad was interested in the spaceships I kept drawing and the strange etchings on the sides of those ships. But in all honesty, I couldn't recall having seen such crafts. It was subconscious etching that appeared when my pen was on paper. In the plain light of day, the idea of a mission sounded quite lame as well. It was definitely out of character for me; I can't speak for Jay. Nevertheless, the me who arrived back in Manyip was like a little girl. I was plagued by nightmares of a black-caped figure, with a face like the sun, wishing to devour me. As well as this, I was tormented with notions of good versus evil. I had trouble sleeping. I was so petrified that at the age of twenty-eight I had to sleep in bed with Mum and Dad.

A trip to the dentist bought up flashbacks of being strapped down and a blue laser light probing my body. I couldn't make out those who surrounded me, but everything was metallic gold, and I had memories of not being able to move. Shortly after that experience, I read Whitney Schreiber's book *Communion*, which was all about alien abduction. I got through the first few pages of his abduction account, and I lost it. His story of alien abduction and missing time were identical to my experience, yet I refused to accept his line of reasoning.

What I wanted was answers. What had happened to me? Was it God? Was it aliens? Was it madness? Why me?

12

The Psychologist

The first thing I recall about the psychologist, Susan, was her enormous red-framed glasses. Susan was an officious woman, somewhat cool and aloof. I wrote down an account of what I had been through, which she packed away in her files.

"My trouble is that nowhere feels safe. It's as if the world has faded away and there's nothing that can support me," I said.

"That's hardly surprising. You've had a frightening experience. Everything you've ever believed in has been cast in disarray—the baby has been thrown out with the bathwater. What we need to do is create a sense of safety in you," Susan said as she got me to settle back and relax. Even to this day, the word *relax* makes me tense up. "Imagine yourself somewhere where there is bush land, the sun is shining, and you can hear the leaves rustling. The ground below you is firm and solid …"

I had lots of relaxation tapes. I listened to them ad nauseam, but either I was a slow learner or they didn't work on me because I became quite agoraphobic, which made it very difficult to maintain work.

Over a series of sessions of hypnotherapy, it was revealed that I had always been in contact with extraterrestrials, particularly in my childhood. The hypnotherapy sessions showed that I had indeed been abducted by aliens, and Susan said that she had other clients with similar issues; all of them had a common drive to make the world a better place. Susan suggested I start a support group for alien abductees.

Looking back on this information now, I still feel disturbed and very reluctant to accept these findings as being the truth. Basically, Susan's work revealed something I can't bring myself to believe even now. Armed with Susan's information, I then went to the local UFO club.

The guest speaker at the UFO club, for some unknown reason, was a transvestite with a noticeably stubbly face, coiffured hair, and a masculine voice. She described almost nightly visitations by beings not unlike the ones I had seen. She talked about energy fields and how these beings were able to tap into our energy fields when we least expected it. I was shocked by what I heard, terrified that this nightmare was real after all. I did what every self-respecting person confronted with such findings did: I ignored it and subsequently never went back there again. Instead I focused on the now and how to improve it and my relationship with God.

13

The Now

The now was horrific. I suffered from agoraphobia, anxiety, and depression. The local GP, upon hearing my story, thought I was schizophrenic and treated me with tranquilizers and antidepressants. All throughout my experience, I wanted to, or had the urgent need to, save the world. On a daily basis I had so many questions, such as Who is God? and Is there a devil? As well as this, whenever I was with someone with an emotional or physical illness, I could feel that person's pain, even if he or she didn't mention it—it was if I could sense it and feel it as well as picture it. For example, I would be talking to someone, and suddenly, in my mind's eye, I would see his eye drop out of his head. Later I would find out that this individual was actually very narrow-minded. As a result of my agoraphobia, I became very reclusive and mistrustful of people's intentions. For this reason, I assigned colours to people, with black being evil, grey depressed, blue healing, etc.

During this time I worked as a registered nurse at a hospital the other side of town, which was very awkward, since open spaces would waver before me and leave me trembling in fear. Mum and Dad, God bless them, made up a tape of all the music, poetry, and words of encouragement that I needed to undertake such a journey. It was hard to work during this time, but I needed something to hold onto.

I recall that during every break I had at work I would ring up Mum and Dad, begging to come home.

At the same time I was going to the psychologist, I was also seeing her assistant. She was called Tamara. She did polarity work combined with massage. Tamara taught me about body energies and following one's own intuition. It was from her that I learnt that the imagery I was getting in my mind's eye was my spiritual awakening process, something that can be exciting but is often frightening. Tamara talked of guides and angels available for the healing process. I recall seeing a giant Native American in my mind's eye who assisted Tamara on more than one occasion in her healing work on me. I was so impressed with polarity therapy that I signed up for a short weekend course on it.

Simultaneously I sought spiritual direction from the Sisters of Mercy. I realized now that I was really pissed off with God, that is, God the father with the white beard, who sat on a throne waiting for me to trip up. As well as this, I was angry that there was only one woman of notoriety in the bible; the rest, men and even this one woman, Mary, were bent in supplication. I felt furious and betrayed at all the women's voices that had been silenced. I was annoyed at the God that had summoned me—a God who demanded respect and total obedience, a God who drove terror and fear into his creations, a God who expected me to give up everything and follow. The Sisters of Mercy were wonderful. They introduced me to feminist Christianity, and we worked through a text called *Woman at the Well*. I learnt to read between the bible's lines and listen to the voices that had been silenced. I realized that Mary had been characterized as pious and all-knowing, when she was nothing more than a kid and unwed when she became pregnant. During this time she was frightened and subject to ridicule by her close-knit community. As for the characteristics of

God, I learnt that God is love and not some tyrant in the sky. As to the God I experienced on the mission, that wasn't God. Alternatively, the mission's God may have expressed himself as an omnipresent and all-powerful being in the sky because that's who I thought he was. I still don't know.

It was a few years later, just when I was starting to put the past behind me, that I contracted chemical sensitivity syndrome and chronic fatigue. I guess the extreme stress I was under and the toxic nature of the house I lived in combined to make me terribly sick. I remember working at an allergy clinic at that stage and being told by the doctor there that was absolutely nothing she could do for me. I was beyond despair. I even drove my car up a clifftop to reflect on my predicament. With tears in my eyes, I suddenly put my hand on the gear stick, readying myself to drive to oblivion.

Then a voice in my head spoke. It said, "You feel unwell because you're detoxing from the antidepressants. You will feel improved in a few weeks, when the blood levels even out." The voice gave me hope in an otherwise dire situation. The only choice I had was the voice to heal myself. Was the voice the same as the previous voice that had led me to madness, or was this the voice of my intuition?

PART 2

Aftermath

Special thanks to
Jennifer Jefferies
Pat Lawrence
Kerry Mansfield
Amber Watson

Dowsing through the Dark:

Finding a Way through Multiple Chemical
Sensitivity and Chronic Fatigue

14

Prologue

As if the anxiety, depression, and agoraphobia weren't enough to contend with from 1988 to 2003, I also suffered from chronic fatigue syndrome (CFS) and multiple chemical sensitivities (MCS).

I have since recovered from these conditions, after ten long years. The exact causes of these diseases are unknown. They are thought to be brought on by a combination of viral and emotional aspects, along with sensitivity to man-made products. Of the people who have CFS, 40 per cent have multiple chemical sensitivities (MCS). I had both.

People suffering from these illnesses experience mood swings, depression, anxiety, headaches, extreme nausea, and fatigue (sleeping up to twenty-three hours a day) when they come in contact with an allergic substance. They may hallucinate. For example, when in contact with a substance to which I was allergic, I saw snakes and spiders. My twenty-first century disease was so bad that I should have moved to the wilds, separated from modern living, to avoid the air pollution, toxic buildings, and so on. However, instead of leaving contemporary society, I chose to fight and stay in the city. All in all, I had the condition for approximately ten years. This meant I frequently had to sit outside in the cold and rain or in draughty hallways, away from other people's deodorants, perfumes, and hair products. It also meant that I often had to be carried home because petrochemical fumes made me so ill. I would then need to spend weeks in bed recovering from the exposure. When I was well enough to venture out, I would regularly get laughed at and taunted for being like Michael Jackson, because I wore a charcoal mask in public places.

The illness was really confining. The extreme fatigue meant that I was often stuck at home in my relatively chemical free house, unable to venture far from its confines. I can't be sure how I ever recovered, but I incorporated a combination of chiropractic, acupuncture, and journal writing, as well as dowsing for health by using a pendulum to determine the type of exercise and dietary supplements I should be having. I included energy healing, changing my attitudes towards illness, and increasing my spiritual awareness while working towards my recovery.

Throughout my experiences I have assumed several things. Firstly, there is something outside of me that heals. I'm not sure what that may be; perhaps it is God or nature. Secondly, there is a smart part of me that knows how to heal itself. The pendulum is one of the tools I have used to connect with God, and nature is the pendulum. A voice would often accompany my process of using the pendulum or dowsing; this voice would suggest supplements, dietary requirements, exercise, etc. The pendulum dowses the subconscious for yes/no answers, becoming a voice of intuition regarding questions of which the conscious mind is unaware. The reason I used these measures was because I simply had no choice; nothing else worked. The medical profession couldn't or wouldn't do anything for me, and alternative therapies and my intuition were all that were left. I also adopted the philosophy "what if …." *If* I were to do something, how would I go about it whilst remaining safe, relaxed, and comfortable? This was an amazing and life-changing thought. I went from someone bed-bound, watching TV, and living in constant fear to someone who enjoyed a rich life despite what would seem to be insurmountable obstacles. What follows are journal extracts of my life as it unfolded and became enriched. At the end of my journal, the exercises show how-I-did-it factors that contributed to my recovery. There are many, ranging from practical realities necessary for survival to spiritual enrichment.

As this story begins, the Vicki of the early nineties was rather quiet, shy, and reclusive. She loathed her job. She wasted her time dreaming up new and alternative healing techniques for her clients, such as You Can Heal Your Wound by Visualization, Your Emotions Created Your Disease by Louise Hay, when she really should be doing her paper work. She was obsessed with a cappella and sang four-part harmonies whilst she drove to her clients' homes. She wasn't a bad actor. She did a good job of impersonating the director of nursing. She was rather lonely. She was still haunted by images of aliens. She missed Jay dreadfully, but since that fateful day in 1988 when Vicki left Albany, she had no contact with Jay.

In fact, I was terribly lonely. I was always sick, with every allergy possible, wheezing and whumping, blurred vision, etc. I was also on antidepressants and tranquilizers. Throughout my ordeal, I kept a diary; it was the only thing that kept my sanity. I have used varying excerpts later to describe my experiences during my sickness.

15

Taking the Plunge

n 1993, sick and disillusioned with my job because I couldn't create an occupation that utilized alternative therapies and spirituality, I finally resigned as a nurse, thinking to become an actress or a writer. It didn't worry me that I had no idea how to do that. I thought that if I took the plunge I'd land somewhere near the mark. A year later, in 1994, I was even more sick with worry, no money, and lots of allergies. I had to re-evaluate my plans. Eventually I gave up my purist plans to concentrate on theatre and began working as a nurse at an allergy clinic. I thought that if I had to nurse, I might as well try to fix my allergies free of charge.

The clinic was run by a well-known environmental medicine GP who tried to combine modern medicine with alternative therapies. This was exactly in line with my way of thinking. I was really quite excited about having the opportunity to see this frontier-type of medicine first-hand. My job was to insert intravenous lines into clients so they could receive supplements and medications that would supposedly improve their condition when other types of medicine had failed. Later, I was to be trained as a Vega machine operator. The Vega machine helps pinpoint a client's sensitivities to particular allergens. It works by an electrode being placed on a special acupressure point on a client's hand. This electrode is able to detect reductions in the electromagnetic field that normally circulates around the body. When someone holds a vial of a possible allergen (something they are sensitive to), the person's energy flow drops on the machine's meter, and he or she is considered to be sensitive. Once all sensitivities are detected, a homoeopathic remedy can be made to desensitize that person, supposedly providing the client with a cure.

16

Twenty-First Century Disease

Two incidents had serious repercussions on my health, culminating with the onset of twenty-first century disease. Firstly, new carpet had been laid in the building where I worked. For several weeks after that, staff members had complained of flu-like symptoms. Secondly, my flatmate, unbeknown to me, had sprayed weedicide on the back garden, and I had unknowingly pulled out some weeds with my bare hands after she'd done that. As the days went by, I became very tired—as everyone does when they start a new job, but this was different. I developed headaches that even woke me up in pain during the night. I also experienced a furry feeling in my throat and on my tongue. I had sensations of being angry, irritable, and prone to violence, which wasn't part of my normal nature. I believed I was dying of a tumour. At the same time, I was reading literature from work about multiple chemical sensitivity syndrome, and the symptoms were identical to the ones I was encountering. I thought I was becoming a hypochondriac and that I was reading too much into it, but as the days wore on, I became sicker and eventually went to see my employer about a check-up. I'll never forget that day, sitting down with the doctor and discussing my symptoms: headache, blurred vision, mood swings, irritability, inability to sleep yet feeling exhausted, and inability to walk far, particularly when exposed to certain odours, like those of new carpet, petrol, rubber, plastics, stockings, and perfumes. The list went on and on.

The doctor told me, "You have multiple chemical sensitivity syndrome. Luckily, we can treat it, with large doses of' vitamin C, tri- salts—which is a mixture that detoxifies the blood and helps with irritability—magnesium sulphate, to help with the headaches and nervousness, saunas to sweat out the toxins, and homeopathic remedies to desensitize you to the allergens."

The Vega machine detected many allergens for me. These included carpets, petrochemicals, rubber, dust mites, and moulds. Vials of homeopathic tinctures were concocted to counteract these sensitivities. I was to suck these sublingually every few hours. I really did try to take them, but when I did, all I could taste was an overwhelming sensation of the substance to which I was allergic. For example, if I was taking drops for carpet smells, I would get itchy eyes and an intense furry feeling in my throat, and my allergies would get worse.

I became sicker, more allergic, and dependent on the clinic for advice. I kept returning there, but nothing seemed to work. By then I was terrified and believed that I wasn't safe anywhere. Desperately I went to the clinic again. This time the doctor prescribed a $700 treatment of a substance called UltraClear. It was to detoxify the liver and the body. She assured me that this would cure me and advised that those who didn't get better were those who didn't want to get better. Meanwhile, I should consider helping others, a sure way to lessen my personal problems. *Sure*, I thought. *How am I going to drag myself over to help others when I can't even help myself?* Whilst on the UltraClear, I had to be on a strict diet of only vegetables, brown rice, and fruit, with no spices, sugar, flavourings, tea, coffee, or alcohol for seven weeks. Before going on this diet I'd thought I was dying, but that was nothing compared with how I felt when I was detoxifying. The doctor said that there were many people with this condition, living alone like me, many so sick that they couldn't get of bed, let alone leave the house. She implied that I was one of the lucky ones. I didn't think so, because I had no one to look after me.

Seven weeks later, sitting in the doctor's surgery, I heard the words that every patient dreads: "I'm really sorry, Vicki. You must be going through hell, but there's absolutely nothing more I can do for you." I wondered what I would do next. I was on my own.

Driving home with my charcoal mask to protect me from the car fumes, steam rising up from my glasses, and tears pricking at my eyes, I screamed out, "God! I'm alone and allergic to everything. Please help me." The road blurred before my eyes. I screamed again: "God, let me die! I can't live in this hell!"

That was the end of my belief in the Western medical system. That doctor was the end of the line. The only positive thing this GP did was to admit I had an illness, called MCS-CFS. Other than that, she gave me no further hope; she abandoned me. I had spent over twenty years working in the system, never thinking that there were diseases out there that couldn't be admitted to or treated by Western medicine. I didn't bother to seek other medical advice, because prior to this doctor I had been to so many others. They had treated me as a malingerer, a hypochondriac, and had talked down to me. I even went to an allergist who skin-tested me and found I was sensitive to many things. All he offered me was desensitization shots that exacerbated the sensation of monsters in my head and migraines. I told him this, but he only gave me some literature on asthma and told me he didn't treat smokers.

17

My Diary

April 1994
Dear Vicki,

I've covered this lovely notebook with special blue, pink, and green swirls of colour and I've glued on a card of two Victorian women with parasols walking along a white sandy beach. I've decided to create a diary and write letters to you, since you are someone I am sure will understand, be kind yet firm if I get too introspective or too caught up in the fear and pain of MCS. I really, desperately need a friend, someone with whom to share my thoughts and insights to help me through this hell. Sometimes you'll be my mentor, my assistant, or my lover, but more importantly, at other times you will be my closest friend. The friends I have are wonderful, but they are only around part of the time; they have their own lives to lead and are doing just that. On the other hand, I am frightened of being left behind, and I don't want to be left burdened with all this misery and fear, and with no sense of direction.

Dear Vicki,
Today was a hellish nightmare.

The doctor said, "I know it must be frightening for you, but there is absolutely nothing more I can do for you." What does she mean?

Where will I go from here? I feel so bloody awful, you know, Vicki, but amongst all this chaos a tiny still voice of calmness spoke.

It said, "You feel like hell because you're leaching the antidepressant from your system; you're experiencing withdrawal." It made sense. All the visual distortions of the floor bending like waves, the increased anxiety, and hypersensitivity to colours—all can be explained as symptoms of reducing my medications. Come to think of it, that is how I feel when I reduce my tablets. Maybe somewhere out there is something that really cares and knows what is happening to me. I didn't feel so scared after that. In fact, I stopped off at COPE bookshop to see if there were any self-help books for those suffering from twenty-first century disease. I felt a wave of nausea wash over me at the shop. It was probably the carpet; I had to rush in and out quickly. The literature I managed to skim through on the subject brought me close to tears. It was so negative and hopeless. I hastily bought some books and am reading them now. They all say, "a majority of sufferers have to live free of the twenty-first century, away from the toxins that makes them so ill … There is no cure, just avoidance of the chemicals that make them sick." It's all so depressing; the more I read the more depressing and impractical their solutions seemed. I don't want to leave Manyip, because all my friends are here. It would be horrible to live way out in the bush alone. Would anyone come with me? I'm going to Jen's; I can't hack this.

May 1994
Dear Vicki,

I'm sorry, friend, but nothing, absolutely nothing, has happened. I'm so sleepy all the time. So tired. No energy. I don't want to sing. I don't want to write. I can't help feeling so depressed. I slept for three days. I'm glad that I don't have to pretend to you. It's such a strain trying to stay calm and philosophical about my condition. I honestly haven't the strength. I feel so raw and vulnerable emotionally.

Dear Vicki,

I expect you would like to know what it is like to be allergic to everything. It means that I am restricted beyond belief, that I am afraid to go out, have no control over what other people do or wear or over my surroundings. Suddenly the world and my home are a ferocious places waiting to devour me. Take today, for instance: I found I'm allergic to even more things. As I was getting dressed, I put on my elastin bike pants. Straight away I felt as if I was going to faint, sick to the stomach, and so fatigued. I had to lie down for an hour. When I got up I changed my pants, and within a few minutes I was fine! Vicki, this house is sick too. It's situated in an industrial part of the city, just down from an extremely busy, polluted road. The walls are stained and the paint is peeling. Everything feels dusty; my throat and tongue itch. The old floral carpet is full of dust mites. In my mind's eye I can see dust mites crawling everywhere. I can't escape it. The high archways have spider webs too difficult to reach with a broom. The house is cluttered with an odd assortment of second-hand furniture. The kitchen has an antiquated gas stove which leaks. You can smell the gas. I need to move into a modern home but don't have the money or the strength. I've noticed the gas makes me sick. The stink fills the air, and I get headaches. How am I going to cook if I don't use gas? I suppose I'll have to keep the door open and wear my mask, but it's an old house and the smell hangs around.

As if the house isn't enough to worry about, shopping is hell. Last Monday I went to the shopping centre wearing a mask, as usual, to keep out some of the smell. The shops were visually bright and gaudy. I had a nauseous feeling in the pit of my stomach. I'd just dashed in to get some meat, hoping to be quick, when out of the corner of my eye, barely registered, I saw someone squirt something blue from a bottle. It was Windex. Almost immediately I felt weak with the overriding stench of ammonia. I was suddenly unbearably itchy.

"Get out! Stop it!" I cried, clawing at my skin, bile rising in my throat and the world spinning before me. I lurched to the nearest table and put my head between my knees. I felt a cold, clammy fist of fear punch at my neck, and the floor heaved in front of me. I closed my eyes, and sweat ran down my face. I must have looked drugged. No one stopped to help me. I somehow dragged myself up and managed to get home. I took some tri-salts to relieve the fierce headache, two magnesium sulphate for the anxiety, and a gram of Vitamin C to boost my battered immune system. I spent the next week in bed, getting up only long enough to pump in more medication and have something to eat.

June 1994
Hi, Vicki,

Lovely one. Nothing much has happened here. It's so hard. I'm tired again. I slept a week, literally, with a few toilet breaks in between. Each time I wake up I see the same old things: the mirror at the foot of the bed reflecting a pale anxious me, the baobab nut I picked up from WA, and a piece of sun-bleached driftwood found at the beach last summer. My eyes get tired just looking at the same scenery. Up on the wall is a black-and-white print of a young woman holding a contented, naked baby. Oh, Vicki, how I want to be that baby—to be held so tenderly, to feel that there isn't a problem in the world that Mum can't fix. I'd like the feeling of warm and sensual touch on my skin. Other times I want to rip the picture up—how sickeningly corny, how clichéd. I want to smash it into a thousand pieces … but of course it's still there, and every time I wake up my eyes enviously wander to that same scene.

Vicki, I am seriously thinking of getting domiciliary care to help with the cleaning. I could get my groceries delivered, too, after last week's experience with the Windex. I would organize lots of things if I could stay awake long enough to organize them. Everything's so expensive when you're on sickness benefits. Why does everything for healthy living cost so much? Cindy's sick too. Her chronic fatigue has returned. All she can do is watch the TV all day, and she's so depressed.

She said, "If I get the allergies again, I'll kill myself." She had that condition for twenty years!

I said, "No you won't. The fact that I'm suffering from allergies is reminding you of those horrible years." It's so miserable here. All I want is some support, and I can't even get it from my best buddy because I remind her of her hellish childhood disease. I need help. We're living on two-minute noodles and frozen vegetables. The one good thing is that Cindy can explain what's happening to me, because she's had similar experiences, and that makes things less scary.

Dear Vicki,

Flat again. Jen and I had a bit of a blue. She doesn't seem to understand that I have no energy for myself, let alone her. She says she has needs. Well, so do I! Bad luck! I'm too tired and my body aches all over. When she touches me I feel like crying. I hurt so much. Even the simplest things are so hard. All I want to do is sleep. I have about one hour of energy a day, and then—*vroom*—I'm asleep. I'm so ill that I feel as if I'm dying inside. Some things are worse than dying. This is one of them.

Vicki, the scariest thing happened the other day. I was sitting in the lounge room reading when I suddenly became aware of the book I was reading. I could taste lead in my mouth, and my fingers felt itchy. I thought, *No. It's not possible, something as commonplace as reading.*

Cindy told me later, "When I had twenty-first century disease I was allergic to print, and I had to wear cotton gloves to protect my hands." Isn't anything safe? I feel as if I'm in a nightmare and I can't wake up.

Dear Vicki,

I'm sitting on the old stuffed sofa in my pyjamas. It's night-time. I'm wearing my slippers and I'm looking at the feeble orange glow from the Conray heater. I feel safe here with the glow from the heater and the TV. I am alone, and the gentle glow scares away the wild animals. Please forgive me for being so melodramatic, but outside, in the shadows, lurk all sorts of wild animals, monsters with fangs ready to devour me. The curtain flaps in the breeze and reveals its rubbery underbelly. Rubber—I'm allergic to rubber. I'm shuddering. My eyes are scanning the room; there's a tablecloth on the table—I'm allergic to that too. I'm now lying down on the couch, looking up at the ceiling. There are large mould spots flowering across its surface. Mould—I'm allergic to mould! I'm feeling fidgety.

I'm sitting up again and looking at the warm orange glow, and I'm rocking. I'm scared, Vicki. I wish you were ten feet tall and these things were wild animals; then you could go after them with a stick and yell, "Piss off! Leave Vicki alone. She's had enough. Don't you come near her or I'll belt you." But you're not and they're not.

Hi, Vicki,

Today I'm lying on the grass. The coarse tufts prickle up through the blanket and scratch my stomach,; the earth underneath feels strong and palpable. The sun is dancing across my back, splashing across my legs, and I am revelling in its warmth—it almost enfolds me. The faint tinge of rosemary and lavender is in the air. The birds are singing in the trees. One rosella, a cheeky fellow, pops right up to my drinking water. For a time I feel free. Not that safe-at-home free, but wild, careless, gaily-abandoned free. This little patch of land is expanding. I'm in the country, and I feel strong and confident. I'm not Vicki, poor sick Vicki, but a strong, capable woman with dirt under her nails. Her cracked hands are rubbing soil together and watching things grow, helping them grow. Lying here on the blanket I'm almost laughing out aloud.

Dear Vicki

I've found I'm sensitive to more foodstuffs. My gut has swollen up like a pig. I have dreadful wind pain and a horrid taste in my mouth. I can only seem to eat rice, some vegetables, and some fruit. I thought it was only a temporary diet the doctor had me on, but I can't seem to go back to anything else. Other food makes me feel awful.

Cindy says, "I was like that. Everything made me sick for years. I spent years in bed just lying there looking at the ceiling. I used to be so bored with my limited diet that I learnt different ways to appreciate a specific food. If, for instance, it was potatoes, I would learn to value the different textures, be it boiled, mashed, or baked, so that I could alleviate the monotony of eating the same things all the time. You can work out what you can eat by the pulse test. If my pulse went up substantially by a few beats per five seconds when I was thinking of a certain food, I would remove it from my diet. I don't know why it works; it just does." Well, I'm desperate enough, so I tried the test with a number of foods, and my pulse rate did increase with certain foods. But gosh, the process is so slow. I'm going to eliminate those foodstuffs from my diet. Hey, if it worked for Cindy and she recovered, why not for me? I also found this really good book. It's the first positive book I've seen on twenty-first century disease, and it's called *Chemical Free Living*. The book talks about natural therapies that are helpful and how to avoid using man-made substances such as petrochemicals, toxic sprays, plastics, pads and tampons, by substituting natural products. It also talks about common foodstuffs that cause problems, such as yeasts, sugar, tea, coffee, alcohol, wheat, dairy products, nightshade varieties such as potatoes and tomatoes. I'm taking all this on board. It's given me some hope.

Hi, Vicki,

It's great to hear from you. I had a really special time with Jen the other night. She looked gorgeous, the way the light shone off her glossy dark-brown hair, the sparkle in her mysterious hazel eyes, and the way her brow furrowed quizzically as if in surprise.

She said, "Hello, magical woman."

I said, "You look lovely," and leaned down and kissed the softness of her neck. She was dressed in her red satin shirt and blue jeans. How I love her! We went outside to stand and look at the moon. It was full bodied and round. We lit a crackling fire and looked at the red embers and we sang. Jen played the fiddle. Its haunting tunes filled the air. We then began a conversation about "penduluming" or dowsing.

I said, "I find the pulse test to be good, but it takes ages to do."

She said, "You could use dowsing to get a quicker answer."

"What's that?" I asked.

"You hold a string with something tied on the end to form a pendulum. If it rotates one way it's a yes, if to the other, it's a no."

"But you're making it swing that way," I protested.

"No, I'm not. I let my mind go free and relax my hand. It's involuntary," said Jen. Until tonight I had seen it as a sweet idiosyncratic thing she did because she was into alternative healing and the pendulum helped her make important decisions. Could it work for me? Could I quickly determine the foodstuffs that caused my allergies? What's more, could it help with more important decisions? I relished the thought of something outside me, bigger than myself, which could help me make significant decisions about something that I didn't have the foggiest idea about. At the same time, I found it a little unnerving.

"What am I contacting when I do this?" I asked. "It's not like my spirit guide, is it?" Flashes of Molhellor and Hector Foyley came to the fore.

Jen said, "It's your higher self, your intuition, the wise part of yourself that you're contacting."

I nervously asked, "How can you know for sure?"

"It's like using the telephone, not knowing the number you've rung, and speaking to someone you don't know. They could be good or bad or indifferent. You feel it. If the answer rings true, you ask yourself 'Do I feel safe?' If you do, then you have contacted your higher self." It seems like something out of a Weeties packet. I'm feeling sceptical, but I am willing to give it a try. "It sounds so similar to let your mind go free," I said apprehensively.

Vicki, I just tried it, and it's as simple as that; it seems to work. I've gotten very excited, because I've tested my foodstuffs and I received the same answers as I did with the pulse test. Yippee! Here comes the cavalry.

Whoa, Vicki, I've found that an inner voice speaks to me whenever I pendulum. It suggests healing techniques. The voice makes me edgy, as it so similar to when Molhellor and Hector contacted me, minus taking over my vocal chords. Still, I have no other option but to follow its advice. Any mention of a mission, though, and I'm pulling the plug on dowsing.

The pendulum brought about an immense change in my life. It helped me make decisions as to what sort of foodstuffs and chemicals I needed to avoid or to take. The voice helped speed up the yes/no answers of the pendulum and suggested herbs and alternative medicines to try that would aid in my recovery. Dowsing became a nightly ritual of checking what was safe and what was not. Jen and I became even closer; we worked as a team. She had a special crystal in a brown leather carry bag that she used. I used a tea bag on a string. When I was unsure, which was often, she would check my answers. The hardest thing I found about dowsing was trying not to influence its outcome by what I consciously thought the answer should be.

June1994
Dear Vicki,

I've found out I can only have a few foodstuffs. Sugars, tea, coffee, alcohol, tomatoes, potatoes, wheat, and dairy are out. I feel so ill I don't care, so I don't miss them. I've tried the diet of veggies and rice for a few days now, and I feel much better, so I will persevere. I'm also using sponges during menstruation. I found that when I wore tampons and pads I got sick and dizzy. The book *Chemically Free Living* told me that these products contain arsenic and bleaches that can make chemically sensitive people extremely unwell. All soaps are to be avoided, except Black and Gold fragrance-free soap powder for washing clothes. All my friends have been alerted to avoid wearing perfumes, deodorants, and strong-smelling shampoo when they visit. If they don't, and they want to see me, they must shower at my place and put on chemical-free clothes. Now I only wear cotton or wool—no unnatural fibres. I don't buy anything new because of the smell. At least I have some control in the house now. The backyard is the safest space, and consequently I spend most of my waking time there. It is so big and full of trees and earth and veggies. I can even have a fire out there in winter.

Hi, Vicki

Why does everything I love have to be taken away from me? I can't eat anything I like, and I have to wear only natural fibres. Also I can't do the things I used to do. There is so much loss, so much grief, and I'm scared, Vicki; if I really allow myself to feel it all, I'll drown in it. Sometimes I feel suicidal, but I just keep hanging on. What if the cure is just around the corner? What if one day I wake up and find this has all been a nightmare? I must be getting better, because I'm whining. It's just that Jen and I wanted to go to a dance. Be romantic, like other couples. I tried, really I did. We went to a "pocket women's dance." It was full of smoke and perfume. I wore my mask. I tried to concentrate solely on Jen, but I felt like an idiot because everyone stared at me. I could feel their eyes and look of revulsion when I came near them. I could imagine their questions: "Does she have AIDS? Can you contract it? She's weird." Anyway, the stink at the dance was so bad it made me sick and tired, and I had to go outside. It was raining and cold. I stood there, and I could see inside where people were dancing close with their girlfriends. All I wanted was to be held by my special woman, like other couples in love. I had to spend a week in bed for that little sojourn.

Hi, Vicki,

I have finally figured out that this illness consists of periods of chronic fatigue followed by a cycle of allergies. I spin into a cycle of complete fear that lasts for several weeks, and then I get the fatigue for another few weeks and collapse. I went for my first official fitness walk the other day. It was for five minutes! I dowsed to see if I needed exercise and it said yes, but I didn't ask for how long. I went to the beach with my friend Lizzie. I barely made it to the water's edge and I ran out of energy. It's as if my whole body just stops, similar to a battery winding down and without warning. My voice slurs, my movements become spastic, and I just have to fall down where I am. But Vicki, the intimacy was just so special. Normally I'm the joker, always good for a few laughs, or the academic, being very logical in the head and having philosophical discussions. But this day it was just the raw me. No pretence. I couldn't move. Lizzie hugged me. I could feel her firm hands stroking my shoulders. I rested my head on her chest and felt her heart beating. Time stood still. The wind whispered through the waves. The gentle swishing of the grasses, and the crimson hue of the sunset-tinged the sky. I had never felt so loved or safe for a long time. That's it! I don't want much, just to be held, loved, and told everything will be all right. There never seem to be enough hugs when you live alone. All I want is to be really held—to feel safe despite this rotten, stinking illness. That time with Lizzie was special. Friends who aren't lovers aren't supposed to be as intimate as we were that day. Still, I ache for that familiarity. When I'm held, it's safe to relax, let down my terror, and let it flood out. Sometimes at night I just sit and cry in heart-rending sobs for what seems like hours. I get so scared, Vicki. Quite often the crying itself completely exhausts me, and I simply stare. It's those times I feel spent. My stomach hurts from all the sobbing.

Dear Vicki,

Yesterday I watched TV for the third day in a row, and I could actually concentrate a bit! My sister Lillie came over and gave me a lovely card and a book. That night I saw the stars stretched out before me like a glittering blanket. I stood barefooted in the veggie patch, smelt the rich earth, and felt its firmness. For a moment I remembered how exciting the night could be. It's so wild and carefree, full of unknown adventures. I spoke to my sister Marie on the telephone, and for the first time ever I felt close to her. I think she genuinely cares about what is happening to me, but she doesn't understand. It's all strange to her, even though she's been reading up on my condition. It's funny, really; as a kid she teased the shit out of me. I guess I could say I even hated her. She's tried over the years to get closer to me, but I had built an impenetrable wall around me. Tonight I felt sad. Here is this woman who I don't know anything about, and she is trying to help me, after all the snubs I have given her! When I got off the phone I felt like chatting, so I rang a friend, June and we talked about *Star Trek*. I enjoy her company. I had been so caught up in myself that I'd forgotten the niceties of the world. We had a good, ordinary natter. Afterwards I went out to the back garden and planted some seeds.

Dear Vicki,

Today I was tired, but I still felt better than I have in a long time. I had a shower without soap and only a little squeeze of baby shampoo. I'll be damned if I don't use *something* to clean my hair, no matter how bad my allergies get. Even though I dowsed to see if I was allergic to the shampoo and it said I was, I won't let my hair hang greasy. Then I went outside. There I noticed a gum tree in the front. In fact, we have two. I'd never before taken the opportunity to admire the exquisite patterns of the bark. I pressed my ear against the smooth, milky skin of the tree, hoping to listen to its breath. I could hear the rattling of the xylem and the phloem (the plant's sap) flow along the length of the tree. It felt so alive.

Tonight Jen and I lit a fire in the backyard. It rained, and I wore my black *japara*. The rain formed beads on the hood, and I remembered a much younger Vicki who used to stand in the rain in her white parka. She listened to the sound of the rain running over her warm comfy coat and knew that she was safe. That's how I felt tonight. Jen was looking beautiful in the firelight. I enjoyed her company. Her touch was so delicate; for once it didn't hurt me, and I delighted in her stroking me. Tonight I'm reminded how much we have in common and how much I love her. We can talk for ages—deeply, intensely, passionately—about how we want to save this planet, what we want to do with our lives, and why we are here. We'd talk about our all-consuming passion for music and healing. Sometimes we are so intense we'd forget exactly what we had been discussing for so long the night before. How I love those times. I want them back.

18

Backyard B Lists

F or me, the only place that was really safe and where I could be myself and relax was in the garden. It is there I could dream and imagine. I loved the outdoors, and in my garden there was nothing toxic. I discovered flowers and held vision quests, soirees, and parties. I never really became a gardener; I was too absentminded for that, but for a while the garden was my world.

July 1994
Dear Vicki,

It's going to be my birthday. Should I have a party? Some birthday this will be—no alcohol, no perfumes, no sugar, no smoke, etc. The pendulum says yes. So buck up, Vicki; let's look at what you can do rather than what you can't do. Okay? Invitation list: Lizzie and Mary, Fran and Tas, Anna and Ollie, Abbie, Cheryl and Kerry, Cindy and, of course, gorgeous Jen. Ideas: Bring chips, soups, and baked potatoes; stir-fry fish. No perfume, no hairspray, no strong soaps. Bring a story to read or a song to sing.

Dear Vicki,

The party was fantastic! Like one I haven't had before. Everyone was so real, so honest. There was none of that pretentious shit of "Oh,

I do this" and "I do that." Jen brought her fiddle. I played my guitar a bit, and everyone brought a story, either that they'd made up or that they enjoyed reading. We set up the backyard veggie patch as the entertainment area. We brought out the lounge chairs and had a roaring fire. A bedside lamp was used for ambience. Some of us sat on the couch whilst others sat on the bare earth. We all lounged over one another. It was so comfortable. We told stories, sang songs, and ate our fish (I normally hate fish!), potatoes, and chips and drank water. All the while I had this warm glow inside, like being a small child and really feeling like I belonged– something I didn't really feel as a kid.

People stayed until about midnight. That was enough for me, because I was really tired. What I found really wonderful was when I was asked to sit in the middle whilst all the others told stories of how they met me and why I was so special to them. It's the first time I'd heard people say such lovely things about me. I was raised in the culture of insults; the more you were liked the more insults you got. So that night, to me, remains a highlight, and my heart was full. I felt lucky that I had attracted such good friends at a time when I couldn't rely on my personality or health. By *not* displaying my usual acerbic, funny traits, I had actually attracted the very people I had been longing to know but had failed to meet when I was well.

Hi, Vicki,

One of the presents I was given was a puzzle. How I hate puzzles! They're so frustrating. But this one was really rather cute. It had cartoon sea creature characters with brilliantly coloured fish, large lobsters, sea anemones, and starfish swimming about an ancient galleon. Nevertheless, puzzles are like my life—nothing seems to fit. In fact, they are so frustrating that at times I want to bang them together and make them fit. *What the heck*, I thought, *I've plenty of time. So what if my brain can only concentrate for as long as a goldfish remembers?* I started the puzzle, and immediately I wanted to hurry up and have it finished quickly. However, one really needs to take time to do this, since the creation of a puzzle is like life: enjoying the small intricacies, the tiny successes and failures of seeing the pieces come alive and take shape. By hurrying I forgo the pleasure of contemplation; that day I remember being so despairing. I had fallen into a deep hole, and I desperately wanted to make sense of what was working for me in my life. I literally prayed to God, asking her to make sense of this mess I called my life. Shortly after this, I had a revelation. What if the creatures in the puzzle scene represented important people in my life? Particular types of sea creatures might represent the gifts they bring into my life. With this in mind, the scene went something like this: My acupuncturist is my anchor. She keeps me attached to reality. Jen is the lobster—bold, wild, protective, yet soft, able to stand up for me and never give up on me. Cindy is the large bright starfish that acts as the guiding light. She attracts my attention; she's been there before me and tells me about CFS and MCS. She guides me through the fear. Me? I'm the small pearl trout, frightened, hiding under a rock. However, when I look carefully, I can see all these other sea creatures around me there to protect me. It's as if my recovery has already been orchestrated by some grand design, and the pieces would fit together in their own time if only I have the patience to really look at what is happening to me. After that I didn't feel so alone but rather lucky to have the friends I do have.

Dear Vicki,

I'm dowsing every day now, with the help of Jen to confirm the findings. It's so much easier to make decisions this way. Should I go out? Can I make things safe? Is that food safe for me to eat? In fact, if I do go to the shops, I covertly hide the pendulum as I swing it over the foods I'm about to buy. It's a wonder that I haven't been suspected of shoplifting, because l look pretty suspicious crouched over the food, furtively fumbling away. In the health food shop they told me that danglers (dowsers) are quite common. In the past I had never noticed people nonchalantly swinging their pendulums over food. It conjures up a funny image, doesn't it?

Now I could nod my head at these people and say something like, "Are you allergic to many foods?"

Hi, Vicki,

Today I went to the park. I sat under a tree and looked at the row of beeches and thought of proud, wild Massai warriors. The wind was fresh. I felt wild and free. I allowed my imagination to take me to the plains of Africa and dance with the tribes' people. Later that day I went to our garden and shovelled the ashes from the party's fire into the flowerbed. I wanted the ash to help the silver beet. A party with such good vibes couldn't help but produce abundance. Some of the plants looked sad, I wasn't watering them—funny about that! I gave them a good water, and they've picked up considerably. There are *liliums* growing in the trough. I also planted cosmos yesterday. The backyard is becoming a riot of colour. I can't believe it, as I have two black thumbs. Despite that, the garden is coming along. It's weird, really. I've never been into gardening before. I actually enjoy getting down and dirty.

I created a Native American medicine wheel today. I find these circles to be really special and spiritual. They seem to connect me with the land and spirituality, the specialness of the world even right here in my own backyard. As I did this, I felt myself to be an old, plump Native American woman with greying plaits. I smudged myself with rosemary and lavender leaves, wafting the smoke over my body to cleanse my energy. Next I put stones in the four directions, representing earth, air, fire, and water. Then I smudged the circle, asking Spirit to make the space safe and special. Finally I invoked the four directions and stood in the centre and prayed. I had my own mini vision quest in the backyard. As I did this, I could feel myself becoming stronger and more focused. A chant came to mind:

> Words of wisdom are like the rain
> They fall to the earth,
> Are soaked by the soil,
> Give nurturance to the plants.
> The plants revel in the rain
> And revel in its melodic strumming.

I spent several hours just sitting there in quiet contemplation. I wrote in my journal and asked God for guidance, asking why I had to struggle so much! As I did this I saw an ant struggling with its load. I thought about what ant medicine represents in the Native American wisdom book. It was all about patience and realism—"what is yours will come to you"—a showing, a trust that the universe will provide in its own time. Sure enough, this little ant that looked as if it was going to bust a gut was joined by a legion of other ants to help it on its way. So I'm not alone. The trick is not to struggle unnecessarily. I spent the rest of the day experiencing and enjoying the minutest details of my circle. Consequently the day slowed down. I could hear, smell, and see the vastness of my backyard, and I was in awe.

Dear Vicki,

You'd be very proud of me. I'm being practical and trying to help myself out of financial difficulties. I'm trying to be enterprising.

I'm very low on money at present, and I've decided that I could make smudge sticks for room cleansing and self-purification. I made forty dollars' worth. Smudge sticks are used by indigenous people to cleanse negative energy and are made of sage, rosemary, lavender and, in Australia, eucalyptus. I perform a little ritual to each plant, asking it to give itself for ceremony. I usually do this at full moon, when the plant is at its strongest. Afterwards I tightly bundle the herbs with string, wait a few weeks for it to dry, and then retie it. I've sold about thirty dollars' worth so far.

Dear Vicki,

Tonight I'm listening to Gregorian chants, which somehow make me feel calmer. As I listen to the music, I'm looking at my aquarium and my two tortoises, Bonopo and Tirapo. I remember how much pleasure I used to derive from them. They are growing so big now, and Bonopo keeps trying to boss Tirapo around. I like watching them swim in the warm green water and seeing them looking like astronauts walking in space. Once in a dream, I was a tortoise journeying among the ocean's green waters and lacy foam. I felt an incredible sense of freedom, sexuality, wildness, and spirituality, all at the same time. I sensed the lids of my eyes sliding over glassy eyeballs. Next I made a slow, cumbersome walk up the sand to lay my eggs. I experienced the coarseness of the sand as I dug away at it with my flippers. As I laid the eggs, the sensation was orgasmic, like nothing I, as a human, have ever felt before.

Unfortunately my tortoises are now a nuisance. Their aquarium is dirty all the time, and they always seem to need feeding. I don't think I have the energy left to care for something else. Oh, Vicki, I'm not like this. I'm a nice person.

Dear Vicki,

I feel so powerless, so in need, so useless and out of control. I have no money, no job, and no prospects. I'm finding it hard to watch my friends succeed while I'm sitting on the sidelines. How did I become so mean? What is my future? Can't I have dreams? At times I feel really bitter. I remember going to a party and standing around reflecting on the joy in our lives, and nothing came to mind. As I stood amidst a circle of women, I was asked to wish one of the women some happy thought, but honestly, Vicki, I had nothing to give. I burst into tears and ended up going off alone and walking around the block by myself.

What do you call a bear without an ear? Answer: B. Why is the sea wet? Answer: Because the sea weed.

Honestly though, Vicki, it's hard. I just want to get well, have my own life, instead of one dictated by illness. I have so many ideas on how to heal. There's co-counselling for my emotions, there's dowsing, and Bach flower remedies, which release emotions thought to create disease. There's acupuncture, dietary rotation, spirituality, chemical-free living, meditation, prayer, and the list goes on. I feel lost. There must be some sort of sequence so I don't burn myself out trying everything. At present I feel as if I'm stretched out in a hundred different directions.

August 1994
Dear Vicki,

I rang Mum and Dad. I felt like I needed some love. Because I'm so tired and scared, I went up to their caravan park. Mum and Dad try, but they just can't grasp the fact that I'm sensitive to man-made products. I remember when Mum and Dad came to pick me up, Mum was wearing perfume.

When I pointed out to her that I was allergic, she only looked at me sheepishly and said, "Oops, sorry." Then I think, *Come on, Vicki, it's just a dab of perfume. The trip's only an hour; you're a hypochondriac if you can't put up with a tad of perfume.* However, sure enough, after a little while of pretending, it didn't matter. A little way into our trip, I wanted to drive the car into a brick wall. The fumes from her perfume were so strong they affected my moods to the point where I felt suicidal. The stench was so overpowering I just wanted to die, so I suddenly slammed on the brakes, flung open the door, and threw Mum out into the middle of the traffic. Luckily Dad was following us, and he picked Mum up. For the rest of the day I was a wreck and had to sit outside on the draughty veranda. I couldn't go inside because their house is so toxic to me.

Then an amazing thing happened to me. I met a guy who said he used to suffer as badly as I did, but after seeing a chiropractor named Andrew, he was well on the road to recovery. I was very interested in what he had to say, if a little sceptical, but proof of the pudding is in the eating, and the guy appeared fairly healthy to me. Dad was so convinced by this fellow's improvement in health that he said he'd take me to see Andrew and even pay for the consultation! So we made an appointment, and we're going.

19

Me and My Body

When I left the environmental GP, I told her that I was considering seeing a chiropractor who was having some success with MCS. The doctor told me that she was seeing him too. I remember thinking at the time, why had she tried to convince me she could cure me when she herself needed alternative medicine! Nevertheless, I had nowhere else to go. A couple months later, I decided to give the chiropractor a try. Previously, if someone had told me a chiropractor might hold the key to recovery, I would have been really surprised. I thought they cracked bones, put backs in shape, and sometimes did strange things with vials, supposedly to desensitize people from allergies. I'd seen a chiropractor for years, and he never seemed to do anything miraculous. But I didn't think *No!* I couldn't think too much. Perhaps Andrew was the opportunity to find my way out of this hell. After all, I had the testimony of a fellow sufferer, albeit an unknown one. So I went to Andrew. Andrew was an exuberant, bouncy man, optimistic to the point of being almost sickening at times. He explained body order (BO—unfortunate name, isn't it?). It made sense. I expected a cure in about three to six months but it was several years before I started to improve noticeably.

Andrew's body order provided the sense of direction I so desperately craved to help me find a way through the maze of self-help therapies, medical treatments, and natural therapies. The theory is that the body has a need for order so that it can recover and remember how to heal itself. The body has its own general predisposition towards healing itself. That is, it can heal or remember to recover if it is done in the right sequence. By muscle testing, a procedure that works on the same principles as dowsing, one can determine in which percentage of BO one's body is. If the BO is maintained in the high nineties, the body is said to be in BO, and the chiropractor, along with the client's intuition, work together to maintain that state.

Andrew acted as my coach. He determined in what order my holistic care should come, which he ascertained by muscle testing. Should I concentrate first on the body (using exercise, chiropractic adjustment, dietary supplements, acupuncture, and homeopathic medicines, etc.) or the mind (in the form of reading, studying, or emotional counselling)? Should the spirit take priority (using religion, ritual, prayer, meditation, joy, following life goals, etc.)? Once the order and type of holistic care was ascertained, I tackled the most important thing and did it.

The ideas for my holistic care, that is, which things needed to be addressed, came from my research, my intuition, and from Andrew. I would also go to other health-care professionals if BO indicated that I needed their care as well.

Andrew no longer does muscle testing. Instead he relies solely on chiropractic, but I believe that, for me, the dowsing still contributes to finding a way through the maze. At the end of this book I have shown how people can do this for themselves. All they need to do is to work in conjunction with a good chiropractor.

August 1994
Dear Vicki,

Today I finally went to see Andrew. How did I feel? I felt more hopeful. Maybe there was a way out of this after all. At Andrew's office, a dour-faced, officious-looking woman greeted us at the reception desk. She had honey-blonde hair tied back in a severe bun.

She looked over at me through black-rimmed glasses, handed me a clipboard, and asked, "Can you fill in these details, please?" The waiting room was full, but Mum and I managed to squeeze in between two women. As I filled out the forms, I could hear voices spill out from Andrew's rooms. *Not very private*, I thought. I looked around the waiting room at the clients. I noticed two separatist lesbians. *Of all the luck*, I thought. *This guy must be fantastic for* these *women to go and seek treatment from a man*. As it turned out, the red-headed woman with three stout whiskers emanating from her chin was a feminist separatist. I reminded her that we had met at a lesbian intimacy course some six months earlier. After the recognition, she became really chatty, but I had difficulty concentrating because I couldn't take my eyes off those large curly hairs jutting from her chin.

Finally, to increase my attention span, I got up enough courage to ask, "So, what brings you here?"

She said, "I've got diabetes. If I don't get it under control, I'll have to go on insulin."

In surprise, I replied, "Wow! I didn't know you could choose to go on insulin. I thought you had no choice."

"Not if I can help it," she said with a smile. "Andrew's helping me through it with BO." As she said this, she had a faraway look on her face, as though she'd been brainwashed.

I wondered, *What have I gotten myself into?* Before I could ponder this worrying question any further, I was called into Andrew's office.

Vicki, Andrew was nothing like I expected. He was a late thirtyish- something with a cheery disposition. He had a red fuzz of hair that hung like a lampshade around his bald head. He wore a bow tie that looked as if it should light up and twirl around or, at the very least, squirt water at unsuspecting people. At the very start I felt at ease with him. He exuded a confident manner. "Let me explain," he said. "I don't cure. I see myself as a coach, directing a patient where she needs to go. Sometimes it may be to other health professionals; it may mean taking supplements or homeopathic. Hop up on the table." While I was there, he asked a whole series of questions concerning diet. Meanwhile, he was muscle-testing me. I held my arm up high, and he would try to push down on it with me pushing in the opposite direction as he mentioned a substance. Sometimes I pushed strongly. That meant my body wasn't sensitive to it, but with others my push was weak. That meant my body was not coping with that particular product. By now I was used to almost anything unusual. He told me, "The tests reveal you are sensitive to sugars, wheat, coffee, yeasts, and dairy foods. Here are some homeopathic medicines that will help build up your immune system." He continued, "Your body is 80 per cent BO. It needs to be in the high nineties so that your body can adjust and begin to heal itself. Until that time, avoid these substances and take the supplements. Your life will change dramatically the more you come into alignment with BO on all levels of the mental, physical, and spiritual aspects. I will adjust you with a chiropractic procedure, and the body will begin to heal and move towards BO." Next he cracked my bones on the drop table, and before I knew it, he said, "See you in two weeks." Then he gave me a clumsy hug goodbye. That was it, Vicki. I'm now on the path to BO!

Dear Vicki,

Andrew was right. I feel so dreadful. Mind-numbing headaches, joint pain, and swollen stomach. I guess I'll just have to hold on tight and endure the ride! I hope this bloke knows what he's doing. Maybe the cure is worse than the disease! I have decided to continue dowsing, as Andrew says my dietary needs will change on a daily basis. One day I'll need a small portion of a particular food to maintain BO, but then the next day I can't eat that substance and will have to substitute something else. It's a bit fiddly, but I think I'm starting to get the hang of it. I told Andrew that I dowsed. He thought it was a great idea and told me to continue. I don't know what I'm doing, really. Also, based on the questions Andrew asked me in his office, I have decided to ask myself the same questions at home, using the pendulum. For example, I ask, "Am I in BO?" If not, I try to determine on what level I need to adjust, whether it be on the mental, physical, or spiritual level, and then use the pendulum and my intuition to determine what I need. Say, for example, I need to improve my physical level. I would list down as many things as I could think of that fall under the physical category, such as exercise, chiropractic, diet, supplements, saunas, acupuncture, massage, and then ask the pendulum to pick the most urgent. It works too. Vicki you are learning so much!

September 1994
Dear Vicki,

Hello, lovely! I'm still going to Andrew's once a fortnight, up the windy hill. As I drive, it's funny, but I get cravings and thoughts of things that I might need for BO. It's as if my intuition knows Andrew is at least going to listen to my needs. Perhaps during the two weeks in between visits I'm too locked in to fear to notice what I need. Or maybe I'm being unkind. The long trip to Andrew's is the only time

I have to let my mind relax and think freely. I still feel uncomfortable with dowsing. How does it work? And body work with Andrew is so weird. It's so far removed from Vicki Weaver ex-midwife-registered nurse. But hey, it's working! Who cares how?

Andrew was right. My life did change but very slowly and painfully. As time wore on, my life improved and the experiences I had were wonderful, despite having MCS-CFS. My disease became my teacher. It pushed me forward towards greater understanding of life, love, and relationships. It made me more determined to "live my one wild and precious life," without worrying whether I was good enough, well enough, smart enough, attractive enough, thin enough, etc. My main question was how to live my "B list" (as Joseph Campbell, a theologian, puts it.) I had hardly any energy to do things I liked, so whatever I did, I had to be selective. I therefore chose those things that made my heart sing, things such as theatre, writing, social justice, and relationships with real integrity and depth. What follows are excerpts of my life as it unfolded mentally, physically, and spiritually—the people I encountered, the visions I had, and the spiritual awakenings during my path to recovery. It's impossible to separate any one thing that aided in my healing. It was everything, because everything engaged all of me, encouraging me to heal.

Dear Vicki,

I've just had the most amazing, erotic, loving experience of my life. This is after Jen and I had been arguing for some time now about intimacy. I'd been feeling guilty about what sort of girlfriend I am, since I have trouble having sex, and if I do, it hurts. But tonight something amazing happened. We both stopped worrying about how sex should be and acted in the moment. It all started when I was lying on the mattress in the lounge room. Relaxation music was playing, and the dull gentle light of a candle glowed near the bedside. The room was delightfully peaceful when Jen slipped in beside me. She could tell I was tired and that I could barely keep awake.

"Lovely, you look tired." She ran her long slender fingers across my forehead and looked into my eyes. Her eyes were large, chocolatey-velvet brown in the firelight. For once I didn't have the energy to tense up; rather, I nodded and relaxed in her arms. Jen seemed to understand too. I felt I could see right into her soul. We lay facing each other, her out-breath my in-breath, the gentle in-and-out cyclic nature of our breathing. I could feel her warm, sensuous body pressed against mine and sense the thin texture of her T-shirt. Next she placed one hand on my heart and positioned my hand on her genitals. There were no words, just the sense of being loved and held in a sexual way. I could feel the warmth of her breasts, smell the sweet aroma of her breath as she breathed in and out. The long shadows of our silhouettes danced and swayed in the candlelight. It was at that moment I actually had a whole body orgasm. I could feel the energy rising up from my pelvis and bubbling up throughout the entire length of my body. I didn't know it was possible if you didn't actually have proper sex. Later I found out that what we had been doing was tantric sex. This involves living in the moment, raising the body's sexual energies and love, and focusing on sending this energy throughout the entire body rather than keeping it contained in the sexual region, which is how Western sex functions. Wow, it was a fantastic experience!

January 1995
Dear Vicki,

Abbie was at my place today, and she showed me the local paper. It had an article about a community project, a play being organized by community directors Terry and Kat.

"Hey, have a gander at this," Abbie said, pointing to an article titled "Community Play Seeks Volunteers." I almost snatched the paper out of her hands.

"Hey, Abbie, this is exactly what I've been looking for, something exciting to do. They want writers, actors, singers, musicians, and stagehands. It's a play about women's experiences with the penal system, both now and in Elizabeth Wilcox's time. Elizabeth Wilcox was the last woman hanged in South Australia." Cool. I felt sad when I read the article. I wondered what I could do to contribute, since I was so ill. I went quiet.

Abbie must have picked up my thoughts, since she put her hands on my shoulder and said, "Even if you only do a little bit, Vicki." I'm now thinking about the project. Can I do it and remain safe? Can I do it and not get exhausted? Could I wear my mask? Could I take a pillow and crash if I needed to? My mind's buzzing. This would mean that I'm leaving the house, and I know lots of people who would love to be involved …

Vicki, I rang Terry. She sounds about my age and really interesting. I told her about my illness and my requirements, and she was fine. She didn't think I was a kook at all. People's acceptance sometimes blows my mind! I'm going in on Monday.

Hello Vicki,

Fantastic! I did it. I went to the workshop. I was like a sniffer dog smelling out odours. This is the first public activity I've been able to do since this wretched illness took over. Terry was great. She introduced me to the writers and explained my illness.

The others drew away from me, saying, "I know I'm wearing something smelly, but next week I'll go without."

Then, with great aplomb, I pulled out my mask and said, "I guess I'll just have to wear my accessory." We all laughed. I then sniffed out the theatre complex and decided the theatre was perhaps too much of a challenge at present because of the carpet. However, the canteen would be great for writing purposes, because it had lino floors and older style furnishings, less likely to contain chemicals.

Wow! Since then I've been to several of the workshops. They were fantastic, right up my alley. They want pieces of writing about issues affecting women in the community. It's so exciting. We're based at The Parks, miles from anywhere, in a beautiful, modern theatre complex. The theatres are all in the round, meaning the cast are seen from 360 degrees, and the flooring is rich red carpet. When the stage lights are on, I feel as if I'm transported to another world, one of mystery and adventure. Gosh, Vicki, they are so intense. They ask earnest questions, and their eyes seem to drill through me with intensity. One's called Amberian, but I can't remember the other woman's name. Amberian's single, a feminist, and has had experience with domestic violence, whilst the other has kids and wants to write about the reality of child rearing. On the other hand, I want to write about benzodiazepine addiction. I'm going to title my piece "Benzo Junkies." You know I'm mad keen on exposing benzodiazepine addiction, showing how the medical profession gets people hooked, then at some stage down the track dares to say one's a junkie. I have so much I want to say about it, especially after what happened to me because of my ex-doctor. I'm still so angry about what he did to me. It took five years to come off that medication. It was such a painful and scary experience. No one wants to know you, either. One of the times I want to write about is when, on my insistence, the doctor finally agreed to reduce the dose I was taking, but he did it too quickly. I almost had a seizure because of that. I was at work, on a busy round, dispensing tablets, when suddenly the floor started waving and bending before me. I felt physically sick; sweat started pouring out of me, and a cold sensation of pins and needles prickled down my neck. I literally had to crawl to the toilet and almost fell face first into the bowl. Luckily, a voice inside of me said, "Take a tablet." I did, and I was fine a few minutes later. If I hadn't taken an extra tablet, I might have fitted. Bastard!

The writing process is so interesting. We read each other's works and do exercises to get our brains working. But it can also be challenging. Is mine as good as hers? etc. Our writings are not the only pieces being used. Women from the prisons are also having workshops. Vicki, the injustices of their lives—the rapes, incest, domestic violence, and poverty—are incredible. I tell you, it is giving me a fresh insight into women, their experiences, and why some do end up in prison. Here's part of the script that I wrote that is going into the play.

NURSE (*says to patient*). You need more Valium.

NURSE (*says to audience*). As soon as I had said it, I knew I had put my foot in it. But Mrs Spiel had every right to know what tablets she was on. Unfortunately, her doctor and her nephew, in their wisdom, had decided she needed tranquilizers. They evaded the truth to call her tablets by the name Valium, instead calling them by their generic name, diazepam. Knowing both parties involved, I'd say they did it for the quiet life. Diazepam, Lexotan, Lorazepam, Serepax, Mogadon, Temazepam, and Clonazepam are tablets from the same pharmaceutical family and are known collectively as benzodiazapines. These tablets are usually prescribed by busy GPs for people, often women, who have difficulty sleeping, nervous tension, back pain, or difficulty coping.

The nurse walks into the spotlight and tells her story of addiction. All the while, in the background, a faceless doctor writes script after script that spills onto the floor, creating mounds. Next he gets up and swings his golf club, searching for the ball, not listening to the story of the woman who has come to visit him.

Dear Vicki,

The workshops are coming on well; they're not all gloom and doom. I wrote about a special time in my childhood with Nan, collecting mushrooms and using an old paring knife. I talked of magical rings and of her soft, freckled hands and her favourite mustard cardigan. We also did a timeline of our lives from when we were children. Now the majority of the writing is over, and Kiersten has collated it into a play. We were given the scripts the other day. Next, we begin the acting. So, what is the story? It begins with the audience walking into what is like a prison. They're all frisked as they enter to be seated. The cast are dressed as wardens. The storyline comprises many women's stories, stretching back from 1873, when Elizabeth Wilcox was the last woman to be hanged in South Australia, to the present. We travel in a horse-drawn box—tiny and dark and smelling of men's stale sweat, urine, alcohol, and vomit— back and forth between Manyip gaol and Elizabeth's trial. The show draws a comparison between women's experience in the past and today, with how they are treated and why they are there. The stories are so powerful and visceral. I can't bring myself to read the script all the way through.

Dear Vicki,

Everyone's involved now. Jen's inspired, Lizzie's getting involved, and Tas's doing stage-managing. It's great that all my friends are working together on this project. I've learnt about boundaries too. I've had to set my limits, rest when I can, and wear my mask when we're inside. It's hard, because I want to do everything, but my body won't let me. Everyone's so terrific. We start rehearsals soon. Guess what? They are going to use all my pieces! And … and I've decided to act. I don't know how I'll cope, but I've just got to do more.

Hello Vicki.

Jen and I have been talking, and we reckon that the theatre space will be full of untold sad stories from women both alive and dead. Many of these stories will be from women of broken spirit, who are angry, defiant, etc. We thought it would be great if the acting space was smudged. In that way we could honour those stories, giving them a voice in a sacred space created just for that purpose. The reason we would do this is because after a rehearsal everyone feels so depressed and full of pain. By creating a special forum and paying our respects to these stories, the spirits can be put to rest. Anyway, we suggested this idea to Terry, and she loved it. Shar, the Aboriginal dance teacher, said her people smudge with eucalyptus, and it's important to be respectful to the deceased ancestors and elders. First we ran the smoking smudge stick (comprised of smouldering dried eucalyptus and herbs) around our bodies as if dressing ourselves especially for a particular occasion. The stick would then be passed around the circle from one person to the next. Next, someone would trace the outline of a circle around us, dispelling negative energies. After this we would ask permission from the deceased Aboriginal ancestors to tell their stories and pay homage aloud to all women, both past and present, who experienced injustice. Quite often we sing a song of welcome. So now we do it every day before performances, and it seems to work, since we don't go home feeling depressed. The cast love doing it, and if we forget, they attribute any bad luck or feelings of negativity to our not smudging.

Dear Vicki,

I'm having so much fun with the cast. I've taught them about the wonders of the pendulum.

"Right." I said, "Let's put it to the test. We'll try the pokies." So we all went out to the pokies with our pendulums, which were actually Lipton jiggler tea bags, and dowsed the machines. We must have looked a bunch of whackers, all crowded around the machine, intently watching the dangle of a tea bag. We didn't care—we won ten dollars! Hey, it's a start.

Dear Vicki,

I'm so happy! Cindy and I have decided to move to a healthier place near the sea; a more modern, less toxic place. It's at Fran's house. It has internal heating, wooden floors, and everything! Mum and Dad said they would help us shift.

Dear Vicki,

We have moved! It's much smaller than our last place, and I'm exhausted. Today, while I was pondering, I thought of two photos I have of dingoes. In one picture a dingo is looking dignified, sitting on a rock. A wire fence breaks the bottom of the scene. The viewer can feel the harsh reality of confinement and entrapment.

The second photo is of a dingo family, a mum, a dad, and frolicking pups. The light is shining through the long grass. There is lush bush in the background. Seeing this photograph, the viewer is transported to a time when dingoes travelled in packs and there was plenty of food. The two photos were of the same compound but taken from different perspectives. The second photo was taken through the gap in the wire mesh. These dingoes, although entrapped, seem to have minds and spirits that are free and have been able to retain their dignity no matter how small their enclosure. That's how I want to be. My body might stop me, but my mind and spirit are endless. How do I achieve this, though? Tomorrow I want to start by noticing a little around me. Perhaps an early morning walk, the fresh sea breeze, an herbal tea at Babette's, maybe read the paper, and I'll start the day with an omelette and a freshly squeezed orange juice.

February 1995
Dear Vicki,

I can't believe it. The new house is a death trap! I should have dowsed before I chose to move in here. The next-door neighbours are renovating, and the smell is wafting over to our side of the maisonette. I feel so sick; nowhere is safe, and now I'm so allergic even the smell of the powder the next-door neighbour washes her clothes in makes me feel sick. The gas from the central heating also bothers me. I was so ill I couldn't stay at my new place. I felt like a fleeing refugee; I had to stay at a friend's house because of the danger lurking at home. It is unsafe there as well, but nowhere near as bad as mine. I'm frightened that my illness is getting worse. I remember the one and only time I went to the chemical sensitivity support group. A woman there, after surviving the disease for twelve years, living all alone in a caravan, told the story of how she had decided to drill a hole in her van to hang up a photo. The stuff that came out of the wall was so toxic to her that it sent her sensitivities into chaos, and her illness became as bad as when she was first diagnosed. I remember the look of fear, horror, and helplessness in her eyes that day as she told her story. I literally ran from the meeting. I couldn't face what lay ahead of me. I'm scared, Vicki. I don't have any money, nowhere to live, and my allergies are spiralling even more out of control. I'm applying for emergency housing, but where can I live until then? It's only a short-term solution staying at Mary's, because her house makes me sick too. Please, God, I don't want to end up like those other twenty-first-century-disease people having to live on Kangaroo Island. I need somewhere with wooden floors, no gas, not newly painted, and far enough away from toxic neighbours.

Dear Vicki,

I've been really practical, gathering information about emergency housing. I didn't know that even if I am accepted, the wait could be up to three months or so. I'm not even thinking of that. Firstly I need letters from my specialist, my alternative health therapists, and from family and friends. I wouldn't want to be dying—I'd be dead before I collected all the information! Then this information goes to a board that meets once a month. Bloody hell! Time just marches on. All I can say is that I'm glad I have the play to keep my sanity.

Dear Vicki,

It's Tuesday, and I'm at Mary's. The safest place is in my bedroom. Outside the kitchen is a sea grass floor covering. Its smell drives me nuts! To top it off, Mary is painting outside, and the smell wafts into my room. I'm wearing my mask, but Vicki, nowhere is safe. I hope this new house comes quickly! Nevertheless, the weekend was really good. Jen and I are at least talking, and she stayed Saturday night. It was so good to be held. I had been feeling so scared, and then to be held as if I was precious made all my worries disappear for a while. The play is coming on really well. The musicians will be coming into the picture soon. It's been exciting seeing the play take shape. Mind you, the content is miserable. I reckon I'd slit my wrists if I had to sit through all of it.

Dear Vicki,

I had a fantastic dream last night. It was about a woman who called herself Faye. She lived in Ireland originally and was hanged for poisoning her husband. She was of a slight build and had long, luxuriant red hair. Her face was pale and wan. The sadness in her face was extremely visceral. I mean, the look in her eyes seemed to be that of someone who had completely given up hope. She was standing on the grassy ground near stone rubble. The wind whipped at her hair; she looked plaintively out across the ocean, and she sang a song in a clear, forlorn Irish voice. It was the most soulful song. I woke up and wrote down some of the lyrics (Jen made up the remainder afterwards). Unfortunately, Jen was sleeping with me and I wouldn't have been particularly popular if I sang the song into a tape recorder at 3 a.m. I didn't even think of going into the next room. Here are the lyrics anyway:

Chorus:

I'm sick at heart from the waiting,
And this strange land chills my bones;
I miss the hills of Ireland,
And those I've left behind.
I'll tell my story before they come for me.
This is the last night I'll ever see,
And I'm sick at heart from the waiting.
It's cold in here …

My name is Faye, and I killed a man,
In that dreary time at sea.
He was violent and forced me,

So I put poison in his tea.
From the windows of my prison cell
On this cold, grey Sydney morn,
The gibbet swings high and grim

(Chorus)

I'm sick at heart from the waiting,
All my hopes and dreams are gone;
For the bread I stole in England they deported me,
So I wait my fate in the morning.
My daughter died and was cast to sea;
With her died the best part of me,
So now I stand, lonely and buried alive.
It's cold in here.

(Chorus)

It's cold in here, close the lid to my coffin;
This is where I belong.
It's cold in here, lying amongst the stones and rubble,
It's cold in here,
This is where I belong.
I'm too young to die.
It's cold in here …

Guess what? Jen really liked it, and we're going to use it for the play. Jen thinks I channelled this song from a spirit who needed to be heard and who lived in the time of Elizabeth Woolcock Maybe, maybe not, but it sounds as good an explanation as any.

Dear Vicki,

The depth of my friendships has really grown, and the connections are so intense. In the past I had fun connections in a joke-like sort of camaraderie, but now my friends seem so much more real. Lizzie gave me a beautiful poem. I've never had a poem given to me before. It made me cry.

"Vicki," she said, "I want to give you this poem. I wrote it for you. I think you're having a really hard time. I just want you to know that I can see that and feel for you. I think you're really courageous."

"Thanks," I said, barely able to talk because of all the emotions welling up inside me. Somebody actually understands where I'm coming from and thinks I'm doing well.

Lizzie looked at me with her sad brown eyes and said, "Vicki, if you need someone to go with you to the doctor's, I'll go." The kindness of people can be incredible! I'm scared of my GP because she treats me as if I'm an idiot. I only go to her because she believes chronic fatigue exists, and she'll fill out the necessary forms. Even so, she looks at me as though I'm scum, and she always talks down to me. I don't know exactly how she does it, but I feel small, dirty, and dumb whenever I visit her. Amberian says she'll come with me to Social Security too, which is great, because I don't know what to do with bureaucracy. I feel stupid whenever I deal with them. Someone should write a short manual on how to deal with Social Security! I feel as if I've been thrown to the wolves.

Dear Vicki,

I really feel this sense of belonging with the play. Everyone is so friendly and supportive. I feel so strong, that I can do anything. It's a bit of a laugh really, since I'm so sick, but I really do feel powerful when I'm in the play. I smash mud all over my body and rub it all over me, reciting a piece I wrote titled "I am Bold Wild Woman." First of all they wanted me to strip naked whilst doing the piece. No way! But Vicki, I'm glad I got to perform it, because in a way it shows how strong I am, even in my weakness, and that women in their everyday lives are strong and able to endure heaps of hardships. Lizzie said it was a very powerful section of the play. She even thought I looked quite cute and sexy! I must admit I've never before considered myself as a sex symbol.

The rehearsals have been going very well, and there's a party every night. We've built up a really tight bond that will be hard to let it go when the play finishes, but as for now I'm enjoying it. One night I stayed up all night. We had a bonfire on the beach at Henley Beach. It's a gorgeous spot—clear white sand and gentle, lapping waves. The moon was full and yellow. It lit a golden pathway across the waters, and Venus, the star of love and romance, shone brightly. Didi sang her song "Venus" to us, singing her love for Kat. It was a beautiful song the first ten times, but after that it wore thin. "Last one in is a rotten egg," said Jen as she flicked a towel at me. I needed no encouragement. The night was warm and balmy. We ran across the sand. I felt its coolness under my feet. I stripped my T-shirt off as I bounded into the water.

"Hey, watch it. It's cold," I said.

"Don't splash me. I like to ease myself into the water," said someone.

"Scaredy cat," came another voice.

"Chicken. Take that!" said Jen. The moon shone boldly up above. I remembered thinking there was no other place I'd rather be than there. We threw a tennis ball to one another and ducked each other under the water. Tiny luminescent creatures darted in and out around us. Afterwards we sat around the campfire, towels draped around our necks, as we told stories and sang songs.

Dear Vicki,

I haven't talked about Shar. She's a gorgeous Aboriginal woman who's teaching dance to some of the actors. She's part of the team as well. She started earlier this week. I just want to talk and talk to her. I've not known many Aboriginal people, especially one who is so approachable and wanting to teach us dumb white folk about her culture. I seemed to feel this strong spiritual connection with her. She told us many stories about her people. One was how the world was created, that Father Moon and Mother Sun gave birth to the Earth and that each eclipse reminds us of this. The Rainbow Serpent created the sun and the moon, and her journey through the cosmos reminds us of that.

We also danced the Snake Dance. I wanted to continue doing it forever. The snake in this dance was the creator snake. To do this I had to let my mind wander freely and imagine I was a snake. At first I felt silly, so I closed my eyes and focused on Shar's instructions. I started to imagine that my body was long and sleek and smooth. I could almost feel my scales slide over one another as I slithered. My hands were my head, and I weaved as my body swayed. I was a snake! I felt immediately alive, vibrant, sensual—all rolled into one. When I saw Shar do the same dance, I understood she was a snake. I could also see the pretty dark head of hers as a snake. She told us later her totem was snake, the black snake! How cool is that.

"Aboriginal people never say goodbye," says Shar, "They say 'LiLiLiLi,' which is the call to connect the relations spiritually and physically. What we change now we change seven times back in time and seven times forward in time." Imagine what an important role each of us has in changing the patterns of our family. If one person learns and grows, so do our ancestors both future and past. I reckon I believe that. It's happened in my family. A lot of growing up has happened on my behalf. Old wounds and scores have been settled. We have gone from a family who disliked being together to one that enjoys and respects each another. I somehow imagine that my nan has also matured after she died, that she's friendly towards gay people and that she understands why a particular family member behaved in a certain way even though the Church might not agree. Poppy is there as well, beside me, encouraging me to study, to go for it, because he didn't have the opportunity. I am finishing what he couldn't.

March 1995
Dear Vicki,

Finally! Finally I've been given a home. It's only taken eight weeks of hell. Jen and I looked at the place the other night. It's a unit. I think in my head I'd envisaged a house, one that was large and separate from others. This unit's one of six but right at the end of the line, so at least I won't feel totally trapped by neighbours.

I said, "What do you think, Jen? It's a bit small and modern, but the ceilings are self-contained and don't connect with the other neighbours' ceilings, so I won't have to worry if they decide to renovate."

"Vicki, you look sad," said Jen with concern in her hazel eyes.

I explained why. "It's just that I think I had such high expectations. But it really does fit my specifications: wooden floors, electric stove, and it's in a quiet block with just a few tenants." I sat on the bench and said, "I wonder what the pendulum thinks? I didn't test last time, and look at the mess I landed in. Is this to be my new home?" I watched the pendulum, a smashed-up tea bag, as it swung. I didn't want to influence it to swing in a particular direction. I really needed to know. Slowly, faintly at first, it swung to the affirmative position and then it swung clearly to that direction. I've thought about my decision since then, and really, I'd been located exactly where I want to be, next to friends. I have nowhere else to go. I'm desperate! It does have a sizeable backyard, and I'll be able to have a pet.

Dear Vicki,

Apparently, in an emergency, the Housing Trust will pay for one shift, and they did. You have to ask them, though. They don't openly offer it. That came as a great relief. All the girls from the play helped me move. I'm so grateful; I just couldn't have done it on my own. I have dreams, hopes, and plans for this little place. It's mine, and no one can take it away from me. I want to plant a bush garden out in the backyard …

Dear Vicki,

Jen and I are still fighting, but we did call a truce the other day when we went to Berri. We had a lovely day and got on really well. It was a three-hour sweltering trip in a car with no air conditioning. When we arrived we poured ourselves out of the car and crawled under a lovely gum tree. The tree almost felt as if it was bending down to cradle me. I felt like I was being hugged. It was a wonderful feeling. This day was the first day in ages that I was able to let my guard down and relax, what with all the moving and the play ending. I had terrible period pain, and I was in agony, but with Jen hugging me and the slight breeze, I felt at peace. The pain suddenly got really bad, and I began to rock. At the same time, I experienced the presence of a Chinese man superimposed over my body. His hair was tied back in a plait, and he had a droopy moustache and goatee. He had a really kind-looking face and appeared ageless, dressed in traditional silk blue robes. Jen said later that he was my spirit guide.

I don't know what he was, exactly, but he said, "My name is Wen Chun, and I was born in 1574. I am an apothecary, herbalist, and acupuncturist. You need some shiitake mushrooms. They are good for the immune system." I hadn't heard of that type of mushroom previously, but later I came across an article saying they were good for the immune system and were recommended for AIDS sufferers. After he spoke to me, my gut started to ache even more.

"I can do some Reiki on you, Vicki," Jen said in a concerned voice. I managed a nod, and with that she placed her healing hands on me. "I can see Wen Chen when I do this; he's wearing blue robes and has a goatee, moustache, and long plait." she said. I hadn't told Jen what he looked like! What amazing confirmation, Vicki; something extraordinary was happening, was shared by the two of us and couldn't be explained away as simply a vivid imagination. Jen then placed her hands exactly where the pain was. As she did so, I felt a warm tingling sensation and the pain felt like it was literally being pulled out of my body and into the air. I could also sense an incredible feeling of love and relaxation. I immediately felt better. But for the life of me, Vicki, I don't know what happened except that I felt much healthier. I even got some of those fancy mushrooms. They taste really good, if nothing else!

Dear Vicki,

Since I've met Shar at the play, I've been having profound experiences. They sound a bit corny when they're written down, but they are so special. It's as if she has acted as a catalyst, and these amazing experiences, loaded with feeling, have been happening.

For example, Mandy, from the play, who has a lot to do with Aboriginal culture, said, "Manyip is becoming a more negative place to live in since we raped the land by stripping the trees and removing its precious stones, particularly the quartz crystals which are thought to give us positive energy."

I feel really helpless about it all. What can I do? I asked in my mind, feeling just as helpless as Mandy. And do you know what, Vicki? I got an answer about some small thing I could do to fix the problem. It happened when I was down at a street fair. There was a table of native plants, and one small plant that would grow to some fifty metres called to me. It looked as if it was literally glowing with joy at being alive. I simply *had* to buy it, even though I knew I didn't have much space to grow that size of tree in my yard. I bought it. All of that day I was wondering what the hell was I going to do with the tree. At the same time I was thinking I wanted a permanent house and the new Housing Trust place I had didn't feel like home yet. I'd already decided I wanted a bush garden, but I knew that my little tree would eventually be too big for my backyard. So I thought, why not plant it where I could come to visit it regularly? It was then I remembered this special place in the hills, which had lots of crystals. I could plant my tree there. I remembered that trees give off positive energy. So, by planting a potentially big, healthy, and native tree there, I would be replacing some of the lost energy taken from the hills. I was chuffed with the idea. In a way I would be a custodian of it. What an honour!

A bit later that day, in confirmation of my idea, I had a feeling that I was a very tall, dark man who was not Aboriginal but who had just walked onto the shore from the sea with a crystal in his hand. I had it in my mind that I was to walk to the hills with this crystal. I later found out from Shar that I probably had a vision about Yurra Billa, a powerful being in Manyip Aboriginal people's dream time.

Yurra Billa is the protector of the hills, who originally came from the sea with crystals and went to the hills. Shar said, "This is a special vision. You have been given a great honour by the land, something few Europeans receive. It is asking you to help in the protection of Manyip by planting that sacred tree at Sleep's Hill."

July 1995
Dear Vicki,

I held a special ceremony to plant the tree. I asked all of my friends to join in. In that way their loving energy would be involved with the tree's development. The day was wet, and water clung to the leaves. The ground was wet and sodden but we didn't care. It was a good day for tree planting. We walked for half an hour down a steep embankment and stopped at a small clearing. The wind tussled at my hair. It smelt fresh and wet, and the sky hung leaden. We cleared the land more and circled the spot with stones. Next we lit a fire in the hole that would give us ash for the plant. We held hands and sang songs about the land and thanked the Aboriginal ancestors for the honour of looking after this tree. Each one of us in turn stated our hopes for the tree. Sam, the environmentalist, lowered a bag of fertilizer wrapped in hessian into the hole. Next we poured the water and then patted the cool earth around the tree. From where I stood I could see the whole of Manyip stretched before me. I saw the blue of the ocean, the plains, and the city's buildings, and I knew this little tree was in the right place.

August 1995
Dear Vicki,

I went to visit Yurra Billa today. According to Aboriginal myth, he sleeps curled all around those hills about Manyip. I imagined I was crawling down his nostril. I walked on further and I sat before a tree with its boughs shaped like giant hands. The hands were so expressive. I felt an urge to speak to him. As I was speaking, I noticed myself talking to a giant ear, which at times changed to a hand.

"Yurra Billa, are you pleased with the tree planting? I feel uncomfortable talking to you because I'm white. I feel ashamed of it. Isn't there some way we can meet on equal ground?" I strained to hear a response, but he said nothing. He just listened and nodded his head. At times I sensed that there were others with him, laughing at me. Other times I felt that they were listening and nodding at me. It was as if I was understood. It was really a profound experience and one I shall treasure.

Dear Vicki,

Another incident occurred that gave credence to the strange connection I had been having with Shar. It happened the other night when Jen and I came home from rehearsals. We were in the lounge room.

"Did you feel that?" said Jen as she shivered.

"Oh that," I said. "It's a very tall Aboriginal man dressed as a kuditche." I said this as if it was quite common to see a ghost in my mind's eye. I wasn't even scared!

Jen urged, "Ask him what he wants. What's his name?" I hadn't thought about talking to this vision, but I suppose I remembered my conversation with Wen Chun, so I asked him.

"I'm from Lizard Dreaming," he said. "The play has pleased our ancestors. You respect us. Don't worry about prejudices. You were born with them. You are a good fella, 'cos you follow your heart. You have any trouble speaking, tell them you act on my authority: Lizard Dreaming. You tell them." With that he was gone. It all happened so quickly I couldn't be sure whether or not I'd just imagined it. But Jen seemed to agree with what he said. I was relieved, because I was feeling really guilty about my lack of connection to any Aboriginals in my life, let alone doing a play about Aboriginal women in custody, and now this man was saying he supported me and my undertakings. Anyway, Vicki, the next day, when I saw Shar, I told her about my experience and described my apparition.

"That's my grandfather," she said. "Yes, he's a Kudjitche man from Lizard Dreaming. He often follows people home from my sessions."

Dear Vicki,

I feel flat. The play has ended, and Jen and I are still disagreeing. I am so tired. As much as I loved doing the play, it has exhausted me. But something that Jen taught me was energy healing. It's like Reiki. I first experienced it with Wen Chun, and then later I felt its benefits when I went camping with Jen and Cindy. We had such a great time that weekend. We went camping at Tarcowie Gorge north of Port Augusta. The place was beautiful, set in natural bush by a small, stony creek bed littered with round, purplish stones worn smooth by the water. We arrived late in the evening. A fire was smouldering in the fire pit. All we did was put some logs onto the fire, and it and it sprang to life. We put on the billy, and when it had boiled I accidently scalded myself with some of its contents.

I was wincing and making a few sounds when Jen said, "Do you want some energy healing?"

Well, everybody knows you put water on a burn, and I just did that, but the pain was really intense, so out of desperation I said, "Yes, do it!" She cradled my thumb and concentrated on the burn. I could feel a warm tingling sensation like I had with Wen Chun, and after a few moments I could feel the pain literally move out of my body into the air. I wouldn't have believed it if I hadn't experienced it myself. I've since become very interested in healing. How does it work? What do you have to do? Can anybody do it?

Dear Vicki,

I have been pestering Jen to show me how to do energy healing. According to her, anybody can do it. Imagine that white, loving energy, full of healing powers, enters through your head and travels down through your hands. You can tell if this is happening by the tingling in your hands, and the recipient feels a cold or warm sensation. As you get better and more confident, let your imagination guide you. It may give you healing symbols or colours and tell you where to place your hands. It may indicate that there is energy or pain stuck in the body. If that is the case, imagine that you are pulling the energy out. At the end of the treatment, visualize that your head is closed to the light and that you are separate from the one you have helped.

Jen said, "It's not you who heals; it's the energy that's given that helps the other person's intuition to heal them."

Vicki, I've since found a book on healing by Diane Stein, titled *All Women are Healers*. Diane says you can use the pendulum to dowse those areas along the body that have blocked energy centres. These energy centres are called chakras, and there are seven of them, running along the spine from the crown to the sacrum. So I tried dowsing my body and found that my heart chakra (ability to love) and my brow chakra (ability to think clearly and be intuitive) were blocked. I then dowsed where I should put my hands to unblock this energy and concentrated on sending myself healing energy. Immediately I felt warmth and an overpowering sense of love and well-being. This went on for roughly half an hour, and then I had a desire to move my hands to another part of my body. All in all this process took about an hour. For the first hour afterward I felt so calm and relaxed, but then I started to feel anxious and teary, worrying exactly what I had done. I have decided to keep a log of my experiences to work out whether it is beneficial.

Dear Vicki,

I spoke to Andrew and to Jane, the acupuncturist, about the energy healing that I am doing on myself, and they said that my energy levels were much better since I had been doing this.

I said, "But about an hour afterwards, I feel much more anxious."

Andrew said, "You feel that way because your suppressed feelings are coming up to the surface to be released. You see, ordinarily you are in a constant state of fear, but when you have a treatment and relax, your feelings have the opportunity to come to the surface." All I know is that I feel really vulnerable and scared, and I don't like that. Nevertheless, I'll persevere with it, because energy treatments are free, and each time I do it I learn more. I get more images in my mind's eye, which I believe to be healing symbols. I think this is because the symbols change from black to gold in colour when that particular part of my body is in balance. I have been practicing a lot on Jen too. When I treat her I also receive a treatment, because whatever is released in her has an effect on me, so I release energy as well. We have been talking long into the night about how the treatments work, and I've found out they are excellent for treating depression, anxiety, physical and mental pain. I've decided to give these treatments to friends for a small fee. I'm keeping a log of the treatments so that I can learn from them. According to Jen, I'm a natural at it. I don't know how I can be so good at something when I am such a non-believer, but the proof of the pudding is in the eating. I have personally experienced the alleviation of pain and felt depression lift when I thought I was powerless to do so. It has also calmed my anxiety down when I was so tense I thought nothing would settle it. Now, to see how it affects others.

Dear Vicki,

I'm so broke! The pension doesn't go far. I'm making smudge sticks and selling them for ten dollars each. I have decided on the advice of my friends that I will do some part-time healing work. They all say they have had really beneficial results from my treatments. Lizzie and I got together to make up a flyer. It looks really professional. I'm setting up the spare room as a healing room for what I'm calling my Tri-energy treatments.

November 1995
Dear Vicki,

I know I've been caught up with energy treatments lately, but I want to make a success of it. Maybe I can make some money or make myself better more quickly. I went to the International Women's Day Market the other day and set up a stall there, doing Tri-energy. Vicki, the markets were full of colour. It was a beautiful day with a brilliant, blue sky. I loved the exotic smells of the food and the colourful book displays. There were jewellery stalls, fire dancers, and martial arts performers. I set up a little card table under a shady tree, put out my brochures, and charged ten dollars for a five-minute session. I felt really nervous and a bit foolish. What if I couldn't come up with the goods? Nevertheless, what happened was amazing. I learnt so much from the brief treatments that I performed. The women who received treatments said the information that I gave was accurate and known only to them! I found I not only got pictures from them in my mind's eye, I also got fragments of words that told me about that particular woman's life and what was troubling her. The readings I got from those treatments amazed me as to how accurate they were, even though I didn't know these women from Eve. Here are two examples. The first woman looked nervous and edgy. She sat restlessly in the deck chair.

I put my hand on her shoulder and smiled. "So, you want to give it go? Have you had energy treatments before?"

She nodded and said in an irritable voice, "I'm sick of having fuzzy thoughts. I want to think more clearly." I don't know whether she could tell, but my hands were shaking and my mind was full of such self-doubt that for a moment I felt like running away. Nonetheless, I pulled out my pendulum and dowsed her body for energy blockages. It's funny, Vicki, once I start, I fall into a relaxing space similar to meditation. I can concentrate fully on the treatments. I told her she was blocked both spiritually and in her ability to experience fun and happiness. I balanced this and released the blockages by literally imagining black stuff pouring out of her body. As this cleared, I saw in my mind's eye that she was once a slave, unaware of the concept of freedom. After a while the images changed to that of black Africans, dancing, singing, and embracing her. Next I saw a picture of her being sexually abused as a young child. The images were dark, horrible, and scary; I felt sick. I told the woman about the images I saw.

"How did you know? I love African music. Anything to do with Africa, and I go nuts. As a child I was sexually abused as well. That's pretty amazing," she said.

I said to her, "The energy I sent you will release those emotional blocks and bring forward your capacity to experience fun. You will be a bit teary for a while, but then you should have a clearer head."

"Thanks, I feel clearer already." she said.

The next woman was someone I knew vaguely, and as soon as she sat down I started to experience some really clear pictures. By laying my hands on her, I found out that her masculine (right-hand side) and feminine (left-hand side) sides were out of balance. This was represented by an angry Maori warrior covered with tattoos as the masculine side and a beautiful, gentle lubra carrying a bark basket as the feminine side. Balance was represented by the symbol of a balanced scale. I saw an image of a European man dressed in a slouch hat who looked about twenty-two. He was clutching the woman, holding her back.

I repeated these images to the woman, who said, "Yes, that's right. I've been trying to let go of my anger towards my son (European) being taken away from me when I was young. He lives in New Zealand, and he's a jackaroo. I'm going to meet up with him for the first time, and I'm trying to let go of all my despair and anger so I can really be there for him. Thanks, I feel a lot saner now."

Vicki, this stuff is amazing. How did I come to know it all?

20

Kay

Dear Vicki,

I have a crush on a friend of mine. Jen's all into open relationships, and we're not getting on too well, so I told her about my crush. It surprised me that she didn't like it much. Consequently we've been arguing. In sheer desperation we tried out a theory. What if arguments are caused by blocked energy? If so, then couldn't this energy be unblocked by an energy treatment? This would mean that removing the blocked energy rather than arguing about it could resolve the problem. Well, it was worth a go. Jen and I couldn't agree on anything. We couldn't even talk to each other without arguing. So we went to the beach and sat facing each other, holding hands. I was so angry at her I almost wanted to shake her to make her listen to reason, but instead Jen suggested we harmonize ourselves, at least vocally, before we began our energy treatment. Translation, Vicki: Jen works on the theory that by singing in harmony we balance our energies so that we are on the same wavelength, to communicate more effectively. I think it's a bit of a crock, but to appease her I complied. After this we then dowsed on our bodies where we were energetically blocked as a couple. We both concentrated on releasing the negative energy by pulling the imaginary strands of energy out of our bodies. It started working about ten minutes after the treatment completed.

We both started to be really honest with each other. It turned out our argument was because each of us had triggered memories in the other that we didn't want to face. For me it was fear of abandonment, because she didn't want to see me as often as I wanted to see her. Her fear was of my neediness. So the more I wanted to see her, the more she wanted to push me away. We've done this type of energy treatment often since, and it has always worked. I think what happens is that the energy removes the blocks to communication, and once these are released, people are able to see more clearly the underlying emotions that are the root of an argument. This method is much quicker than either counselling or talking about the problem with others. On one such occasion Jen and I found out that we needed to pursue other things and that we should break up.

December 1995
Dear Vicki,

With Jen out of my life for the past few weeks, I've no one to confer with. I have to do all my own dowsing, and I don't feel as confident. I feel damn lonely. There's no one here to make everything seem all right, even for a short time. I realize now that being single means being on your own. My other friends have busy lives that don't always include me. The simplest things become so hard, because I don't have anyone I can rely on to encourage me— to go out with my mask, to help with the shopping, to stand up to others and voice my special needs such as, "Please don't wear deodorants or perfumes or burn incense." Vicki, it's so tiring. Everything is a battle. My allergies are really bad at present. I feel worse because I'm alone in this, and I'd rather die than stay home all the time, even though that is where I'm the safest. I suppose I'll just have to push my way through it all. In counselling they have what they call a "support tree." I thought

I could write a list of the things I need help with and get a friend to organize other people to help out with some of them. For instance, Lizzie said she would be happy to cook me a meal and do the dishes. Lillie said she'd help with the garden. What I need is for a key person to organize what needs doing so that I don't have to get embarrassed and exhausted trying to organize things for myself. I've found friends run away from neediness, and if I give them an option of some of the things that need doing, they are far more forthcoming. I've gone past the point of feeling too proud to ask for help. I'm still sleeping fifteen to sixteen hours a day, and when I'm awake I'm tired. My major problem is how to make friends, when I'm sick and have so many allergies! How do I get the help I need? Vicki, I've found writing a list of my special needs and planning how to achieve this works really well. I've decided to start up a lesbian singles breakfast club. Then I can ask members not to wear perfumes, etc. and at the same time meet single women.

Oh, Vicki, one thing that keeps me going is my crush on Kay. She's just so gorgeous, with her brown eyes, dark hair, and the cutest furrow in her brow whenever she's thinking. We have such long talks deep into the night. We have Catholicism and growing up in small country towns in common. She calls me her special friend. The trouble is she's taken, but I can't help but hope.

Dear Vicki,

I feel so embarrassed. I figured out a way to save a few dollars on buying water by using my big blue 25 litre water container instead of a smaller twenty-litre container. The problem is I got caught the other day trying to pass it off as a twenty-litre container.

"Oi!" he said, "What do you think you're playing at? Some people have all the nerve." He dragged me back to the counter. I felt dirty and ashamed.

I stammered, "Isn't it a twenty-litre container? I'm so sorry." I couldn't even look him in the face. I had to pay an extra two dollars. I wouldn't even have done it if I hadn't been so broke. By the time I buy all-organic food and pay for acupuncture, chiropractic, and the rent I have hardly any money left!

Dear Vicki,

Amongst all this hardness, Kay has become really important to me. We had breakfast together this morning at 7 a.m. Me. Up early? I must be keen! It's amazing, Vicki, how that time of the morning with someone special seems so exciting and exhilarating. Everything she does is just so interesting. We had buckwheat pancakes with honey and lemon drizzled over them, followed by mangoes, banana, and apple accompanied by a cup of herbal tea. It's remarkable how I actually enjoy cooking, now I'm on a special diet and I have to think about it. It's really interesting creating and enjoying the different textures, blends, and colours. It's all such a calm and relaxing thing to do.

Kay said, "Food should be chosen for the vitality and the vibrancy that it emits. It makes you feel happy to be alive when you eat it. Cook consciously with thoughts of love and fun. In that way, those thoughts will be passed on to the consumer, just as in the movie *Water for Chocolate*." She's right, Vicki, I feel really healthy after eating all that good food instead of being weighed down by the stodginess of the types of foods I used to eat. Mind you, Vicki, I am perhaps a bit aware that if I ate cardboard I might feel that way too, since Kay seems to make everything special!

There was a moment there that day when I went to the sink to put a glass away. I stood directly behind her. I could smell her and wanted to put my arms around her. Instead I said, with a knot in my stomach, "Have you seen how many bricks I've laid?"

February 1996
Dear Vicki,

I've really fallen into a hole. It's been three months since I've finished the antidepressants, and after breaking up with Jen I can feel a black cloud enveloping me—literally. I can't bear looking at the colour black, let alone wearing it myself. I also get these intense feelings of anger, which come on like a powerful pressure in my head. The only way I find relief is to rip up paper or bang pillows together. The pendulum says I need counselling. I agree, but when I tried to find someone, the waiting list was for several months, and I can't wait that long. I can't afford private counselling. I just don't have that type of money. I've been hearing a lot about something called "co-counselling." It's a self-help type of counselling. Amateur counsellors take turns counselling each other after being taught certain methods. These tools are aimed at releasing blocked emotions. There is a sixty-dollar course called Fundamentals beginning soon. It's worth a try, because once these skills are learnt and you are buddied up with some counselling partners, it's free— my kind of therapy! I've had a few free sessions already, and it certainly releases stuff. I've been told, according to this therapy, everyone is uniquely good and that we get blocked in expressing our true selves because of past hurts. Co-counselling aims at releasing these emotions so that we can heal ourselves. We release these emotions by discharging (unfortunate term, I think) in the form of yawning, giggling, crying, or expressing anger. There's more to it than that, but that's it essentially. I had a session with a woman called Martha, who is high up in the co-counselling fraternity. Initially I felt really uncomfortable. I yawned and giggled and became acutely embarrassed, but she kept encouraging me to let these feelings go. Vicki, I found myself being really angry. I was banging cushions and being told that it was OK; apparently the feelings behind this were that I didn't think it was fair that I became sick and couldn't do what I wanted to do. I had so much built-up anger and bitterness; I could literally taste the sourness in my mouth. Vicki, it was really liberating to voice my hurts and to ask for the cuddles I needed. Years ago I had a co-counselling session, and I thought it was absolutely weird, what with discharging etc., but I've changed my mind now that I have all these feelings that I don't know how to handle. So stay tuned, Vicki, for the next co-counselling instalment.

Dear Vicki,

I have been trying to do my place up to cheer myself up a bit. I get so bored looking at the same dreary backyard. I want to pave it, to move the clothesline to the side, and plant creepers to hide the ugly galvanized tin fence. The problem is how to do it without any money. Well, I've come up with this idea of liberating red bricks from the community, usually one or two at night, armed with a torch, and not from private residents. This is me, whose only other crime was to borrow a roadside flag for my cubby when I was a little girl, only to get up at 3 a.m. to return it because I thought someone might die because I took it. Oops, that is besides filling the so-called twenty-litre water bottles!

Dear Vicki,

I've found a stash of bricks at an old building site about to be demolished. My friends helped me liberate some today. It's really quite thrilling not knowing whether I'll be caught or not. Vicki, do you think you are opening the doorway to a life of crime? Life is certainly shadier when you can't even afford enough food, let alone luxuries like second-hand bricks. But the thought of being caught as I was at the shop terrifies me. Tonight I feel sick—not with worry, but I think I'm allergic to mortar, because I chipped the old stuff off the bricks without using gloves. Vicki, am I being punished? You can tell I come from good ex-Catholic stock!

I'm still thinking of Kay. I wonder what she's like to kiss properly. She gave me a taste of it today when we bade farewell. Time stood frozen. I saw her smooth brown skin, the contours of her face. I smelt her sweet breath as she leant upward and kissed me briefly, for what felt like eons, tenderly on the lips. Then we held a full body embrace.

Dear Vicki,

I went with Lizzie in a fast car for a quick getaway with stolen booty from a park. Lizzie became nervous and said she felt guilty. She's never "liberated" before, even though I told her what we were doing was liberation, not theft, and that these particular bricks needed to be set free to live out their lives in my garden.

Dear Vicki,

Chipping away at the bricks is definitely making me sick. The fine particles of cement get through my mask, and I can feel the dust fly onto my clothes. I came out with a dreadful headache and had mood swings. I suppose at this rate I'm going to be really old by the time I've finished. I spent more time with Kay today. We went to Magic Mountain. There was a blood-red sunset that melted into the surf. We stood on top of the mountain and watched the sky turn to indigo black. Sea gulls screamed as they scavenged for food. I was acutely aware of her presence—the smell of sunshine and Omo. We had fun. We sat on the boats that circled the mountain. From behind, her shoulders were good swimmer's shoulders: firm, broad, and strong. Vicki, she reminds me of all that's good and safe, of the nice days, of church, of Nan, of being awkward, and of feeling like a nice kid from the country who's come to the big bad city. If I had died then, I would have died happy.

June 1996
Dear Vicki,

Before Jen and I broke up, we committed ourselves to a dream of creating a living lesbian museum installation called *Les Amuse*. Mary, Lizzie, Jen, and I wanted a way to celebrate lesbian lives in our community and what we came up with was *Les Amuse*. This would comprise theatre, poetry, photography, and music. Well, we've found a forum for it at the Lesbian Conference in Alice Springs. So it's full steam ahead with its production. So everything's a buzz. We're arranging workshops. I'm involved with the writing and acting, along with Lizzie, who's had experience.

Jen's in charge of the music and Mary the photography. It's fun, Vicki, but it's also bloody hard with Jen. Jen and I are hardly talking. She's got a new lover, and I feel shitty and pissed off about that. How can she be so happy when I feel so down and I'm single? We've both decided to leave our differences at home whilst we do *Les Amuse*, though. We're all one big happy family—not! Nonetheless, we're doing our best for the highest good. It a bit like trying to have a nice family Christmas. The group, now that we've split up, is much easier because I don't see Jen as much. All I have to do is concentrate on the writers' group, and that in itself is a bit of a challenge, because everyone is so damned talented. I read the material I've written and it sounds so amateurish in comparison. It seems it's not just enough to get the message out there; it's also important to refine and craft one's work. I'm learning that there is so much more involved. After all, the other writers have studied writing at uni and in other workshops. Still, Vicki, I reckon all of us, regardless of finesse, have something important to say. I really want to say something positive about the battle with twenty-first century disease, something that quite a lot of lesbians share. I came up with this piece titled "The Strength in Me."

This will be performed with the speaker being swaddled in paper, and as she speaks, more paper will be peeled off to reveal a woman with a face mask, standing defiantly, strong yet vulnerable.

The strength in me,
Sitting alone and afraid in the house,
Each moment becoming more allergic than the last.
The rubber hot water bottle, the lead print on the page,
The backing of the curtains, the house-dust mites, scents
and perfumes, the sleeping bag on my bed,
The soap I wash myself with,
Some of the foods I eat, and the gas I use for cooking.

The strength in me
As I play Russian roulette,
Never knowing which substance will affect me next.

The strength in me,
Hearing the doctor's words, "There is no cure."
The strength in me,
Driving home afterward, locked in my own toxic hell,
With its fumes
Penetrating my senses.

The strength in me
As I drift from sleep to fear to sleep.

The strength in me
To endure the headaches, fatigue, and muscle pain
Day after day after day;
Waking night after night,
My head held in a vice,
Being battered by a blunt hammer.
The strength in me
to go on, despite my loss of dignity.

The strength in me
to be held by my lover,
Each touch feeling like razors,
My body being violated.
The strength in me
To give more than I can.
The strength in me
To continue loving another,
Despite a meagre half-hour's worth of energy for me.

The strength in me
To bear the loss of everything I love:
The gentleness of a hand on my cheek,
The passion, the bike riding, the walks in the bush,
Songs, poetry,
The smell of living,
The taste of cake, wheat, coffee, and sugar.

The strength in me
Sitting in the lounge room,
Huddled in the corner,
Looking deeply into the blinking eye of an ancient electric heater.

The strength in me
To sit with my sensitivities minute by minute,
Letting myself go under,
Drowning in the fear and pain,
Wave after wave of wanting to be held
But knowing no one could ever hold me that long.

The strength in me
To find my own way out,
To intuit my own healing.
The strength in me
To create safety in a metre square,
Working from that square to the next.

The strength in me
To get out there and refuse the alternative.
The strength in me
To dare.
The strength in me …
The strength …

Dear Vicki,

At the workshops Lizzie has written stuff about her cousin Amy, who was a cupboard lesbian in the country. The poignancy of her stuff and the vividness of her words are so real. I can literally walk in the shoes of her cousin who committed suicide because she felt she was the only one who was a lesbian. Similarly, Julie's piece on being attacked was visceral and equally provocative. The way the assailant crept up beside her and grabbed her with the dog lead; it was chilling. Mine, in comparison ("The Strength in Me"), seems so unprofessional—corny, so self-effacing—but I truly believe it's important to acknowledge lesbians, how they deal with illness, and to recognize the strength in these women to live meaningful lives. For that reason I have decided to include it in my repertoire of pieces, even though it is by no means amusing or my best written piece. What I'm trying to say in that poem is to acknowledge that it takes guts to live every second of the day with illness.

I want to say, "Hey, you out there, with your safe lives. You don't know how bloody lucky you are." If they could only try to imagine for a minute how much courage is needed to go to the outside, where the world is full of chemicals that are toxic, chemicals that make one see spiders and snakes in one's head and cause emotions to plummet. Then they would realize that everything is far from all right and that everyone needs to have compassion and respect for other people's weakness and to admire their determination. I think it is hard for women with disabilities. It's time we, as a community, recognize that struggle, that we become aware of the toxic nature of our world and bloody well do something about it.

Dear Vicki,

Kay and I went away camping for a whole weekend. Separate tents, worse luck! The weather was perfect, and I felt like I had died and gone to heaven. We camped at Tarcowie Gorge, with its gum trees and a purple-rock creek bed. We walked along one of the beds for a long way and sat listening to the breeze, the rustling of the reeds, and the chirping of the birds. A small gecko scampered up a log in front of me. We talked of living in the moment.

"You know what, Vicki? We never just sit and be; we're always worried about what's going to happen."

I nodded. "It's great; today we're doing it. Everything seems so special, as if I'm seeing it for the first time." With that we both nodded and sat down under the shade of a tree.

Kay said, "Vicki, you know Lizzie's piece on Amy? It reminded me of how dirty I feel when I think of sex, let alone being a lesbian." I nodded in agreement.

"I used to get headaches as a kid when I thought I must have been a boy," I said. "I thought God must have put me in the wrong body, because I liked boy things and felt like kissing the girls."

"Amy must have been in so much pain; she would've hated herself."

"I did," I said. "I remember praying as a kid, my eyes squeezed tight, 'Please, God, make me a boy,' but each day I'd wake up as a girl." Kay looked at me then with so much compassion. She didn't have to say anything; she knew what that pain must have been like. I loved her even more at that moment. We both sat in silence, a warm comfortable space between us. Dappled light fell on the creek bed.

"Hey, look at that, the rock over there resting on the tree."

I followed Kay's gaze, and sure enough, there was a large boulder resting on the side of a tree in a very unusual position. They were leaning against each other as if giving support to each other in a loving way.

"You and I are like that odd-looking pair, unusual but a perfect fit. Somehow we fit together despite our differences," Kay remarked. I took a photo of the rock/tree companions, and afterwards I put it on my fridge.

Dear Vicki,

What a wonderful morning. It's raining, and the trees are laden with water droplets. I can hear the sound of water rushing along the gutter and overflowing in tiny waterfalls. The sheets are warm and cosy, and I'm all nestled up inside. I am thinking, "What would it be like to wake up on a rainy day beside Kay?"

Dear Vicki,

One of the women, another Julie, who has come along to our workshops, has donated $250 to *Les Amuse*. She can't go herself but has offered to sponsor me to the conference. That's fantastic, because otherwise I would have no money to get there. The other Julie said she'd take her family's RAV4 up to Alice Springs, and I can go up with her.

August 1996
Dear Vicki,

We're on the road. It's a great car, newish but not brand new, so I don't have to wear my mask. It has quadraphonic sound. I can wind down the windows without being killed by the fumes. The intellectual conversations and repartee are wonderful. The perk to this trip is remembering what it's like to be affluent, driving along in the RAV4, looking down on the old "utes" and vans whilst feeling all clean and smart inside. I'm so excited, and I've spent all my time talking about my crush on Kay. All the while the sky's powder blue, the desert so red, and the vivid perennial flowers poke up their heads from a bloodied sea. We're at a roadside stop now, eating lunch by a galvanized tin rainwater tank. It's almost hot. Just think, Kay's on her way too. Is she thinking of me?

Dear Vicki,

We arrived today. The women were laconically sitting on camp stools. They were wearing their Akubras and tank tops, looking very

Strine and a bit scary. Both Julie and I wanted to turn around and go back home again. Instead, we decided to camp a fair distance from them. I saw Jen; she fitted in with them right away, and she's ever so in love! She seems to look straight through me ... And Kay, she'll be along later, and Vicki, I'm going to tell her how I feel before I explode. I can see her now in my mind's eye. She's smiling, waiting for me to tell her.

Dear Vicki,

I told her—I declared my love for her! It was sunset when Kay and I walked down the white sandy creek bed. The moon was already awake and crescent-shaped. Kay and I walked in silence, hand in hand, cool soft hands, everything feeling so right. We turned and faced each other. She looked at me expectantly, as if she was waiting for something. She was so beautiful, so animated.

"You know Vicki, Mary's really pissing me off lately. I don't know what to do," Kay said.

"I'm sorry. It sounds hard," I said. She nodded and began talking again. Her lips were moving, but I couldn't make out what she was saying, I was so nervous. We climbed a large rock face and sat on the flat of the rock overlooking a valley, sea of red dirt, eucalyptus, and a winding white creek bed that snaked its way into the distance. It took my breath away.

"Here I am going on about me and my squabbles when there's something important you want to say to me," said Kay. The air was palpable. "Well, spill it. What's so important that you have to say to me?" I felt sick. I became restless, and I began to shuffle. "It can't be that bad ... go on."

"I've chosen to fall in love with you," I blurted. *Oh, how corny*, I thought. Silence. A long, aching moment. I strained. Maybe I only thought I told her.

I looked at Kay's face. It didn't seem to register anything. I was about to speak again, when she said, with the most exquisite look in her eyes, "Oh, Vicki, I love you in my head and in my heart but … not sexually."

I felt as if I'd been winded. I couldn't think what to say. How could I have been so stupid, so dumb? Quickly I said, "Then can you hold me for a while?" Then I cried. I didn't want to, but I did. As I sidled up to Kay, I could hear her heart beat through her cotton shirt and smell her, knowing I would never be this close again.

When I stopped crying and we'd hugged for a while, Kay said, "When we get home, I don't want to see you for a month. I need to think about our friendship."

Dear Vicki,

The show must go on. I didn't have much time to think about Kay's response. We had a performance that night. This is where co-counselling came to the fore. By releasing all the fears and inadequacies before the performance, I was able to perform with the minimum of anxiety. The stage was raised and partially outside. There were about one hundred women there. Not bad for a first performance! They gave us several curtain calls. Actually doing the performance took my mind off Jay's response. Mind you, the situation was pretty tense between Jen and I, and between Kay and Vicki, I don't know how you get yourself into these predicaments. Later, several women came up and thanked me for doing a piece on twenty-first-century disease. Apparently there were two or three others who were there who had the syndrome to more or less the same degree as I have. The audience also liked my sexy comedy piece titled "The Bi-Lo Crush," but I felt a bit ashamed about that since, in reality, it was a piece I had written about Kay after our kiss. After the performance we were all high that night, and there was a dance. I had organized with Lizzie that

I would have a dance with her. Unfortunately, I had used up all my energy at the performance and with Kay. When I got to the dance, I wound down like a clockwork toy and ran out of energy. I literally had to lie on the floor. My words became slurred, as if I was drunk. It was frightening. I tried to walk home, but I couldn't even crawl. That was when Lizzie found me in the darkness. She half carried, half dragged me to my tent and there I stayed alone (Julie had already left for Manyip). In the distance I could hear women laughing, having a good time, and dogs were barking. I was spent, and I felt so alone.

Dear Vicki,

I have spent twenty-four hours here, unable to move from my tent except for brief toilet breaks. Luckily I have some packet food with me, as I don't have enough energy to walk back to base camp. Today I found a piece of smooth green glass. It must have been washed up by years of being in this creek bed. I'm holding it up to the sun. The world is green, and it's another world and another time. I'm with Nan. I'm walking with my tiny hand in hers. Her hands are plump, soft, and mottled with freckles. I feel as if I'm ten feet tall, because I'm with my nan. Nan makes everything all right in the world. Now I'm exploring playing pirates and climbing over ruins looking for gold. The earth is hard and compact. I see shards of glass on the ground forming a kaleidoscope of colours. Nan's calling out, "Watch your feet …"

Dear Vicki,

The rest of the camp was horrible. I was so lonely and tired. This is the last time I will do something for an important cause without thinking of the consequences. Really, what was I thinking, when there was so much emotional shit causing tension! On the way to

Alice Springs I had apparently been accused by Julie of being feral. I discovered she thought this about me when I found an open letter in our tent after she left to go back early to Manyip. In it she described me as the feral bush pig from hell! It hurt. I had showered regularly and washed the dishes, so I don't know why she described me like this to her friend. She didn't know the meaning of the word *feral*, because if she had, she wouldn't have described me in this way.

September 1996
Dear Vicki,

I did a letting-go-of-Kay ceremony. I worked with the dark moon, the time for releasing. I smudged a sacred space in the backyard. The sky was punctuated with twinkling stars, and the air was crisp. I lit a small fire and smudged myself. Then slowly, painfully, I wrote down all the things I could about Kay and what I would miss about her. Then I threw the paper into the fire and watched the flames lick it up. The ash was used for the garden. I used scissors, symbolically, to cut my ties from Kay. Then I simply sat and stared into the fire, trying to remember how special fires are to me.

With Kay out of my life for the time being and Jen well gone, I was very lonely. I had trouble with depression, and my emotions were all over the place. Co-counselling and energy healing worked to lift the depression, but what I was missing was companionship. This came to me in the form of Imogen, a pets-as-therapy golden retriever- Labrador cross. Anyone with a disability is eligible to apply for a fully trained dog, but if you have allergies, I would recommend a labradoodle or poodle, as they don't lose their hair. Imogen (Immy) gave me love and adventure. It was with her that I roamed the wilds of The Point to find her a place where she could explore and run wild. It is because of her I fell in love again with nature, even if this place was a mixture of toxic waste and beauty.

21

Immy

Dear Vicki,

I'm so excited I have a dog! She's big, she's bold, and she's hairy and gold. She's ever so dignified. I'm going to call her Imogen— Immy for short. I took her to my favourite spot at The Point, a natural, yet toxic, piece of land that is rimmed by factories; the river cutting through the land looks surreal. I walked with Immy up the bike track, sat on a dirt mound, and hugged her big, woofy body. I could hear her panting and feel her stillness. We both looked at large round pelicans spiralling the thermals, and I remember thinking, *Yes, I'm home.* A poem:

She stinks,
But I love her.
She's got mucky goo at the end of her snout.
Her body is covered in mud and lettuce weed,
Her smile as wide as a grin.
I throw a stick for her, but she prefers to wander.
We walk across the white sand,
Littered with discarded junk,
Past the mangrove trees swaddled in plastic bags,
And I wonder about the fish and dolphins

That sometimes play in the river.
But my dog doesn't care.
She bounds heavily across the beach, chasing sandpipers.
I think of the family of five silver and black-backed dolphins
I saw the other day,
That swam up almost to the shore
And laughed, slapping their tails hard against the water.
They jettisoned from the prow of a passing tug.
Then I set about my task,
Peeling plastic bags from tender new roots,
Plucking and primping at them,
Walking softly
Where they sprout up from the watery sand,
Shoving more
Rubbish into my Coles bag.
And Immy, she races on ahead,
An explorer
Discovering new treasures.
She's round and sleek like an otter.
With a smile as wide as a grin.

Dear Vicki,

I feel terrible. I can taste hair in my mouth, and I'm headachy. I dowsed with the pendulum, only to find out what I already know. I'm allergic to Immy. Shit! Well, I'm not going to give her up without a fight. Here's what I'm doing, Vicki, so that I can keep her. Vacuum daily. There's no sleeping in my bedroom with her, and at my acute allergy time, I wear a mask and cotton gloves when handling her. She doesn't care what I look like. All this extra annoyance seems to be working, since after a couple of hairy weeks I'm starting to feel better, and I won't be giving Immy away just yet. Anyone visiting would see the strange sight of me, wearing a mask and cotton gloves, cuddled up to Immy on the lounge!

Another important thing that happened to me at this time was meeting a woman called Amber. She was cool, trendy, and intelligent. She also had chronic fatigue and MCS. She, too, was disillusioned with the medical professionals who had offered her no relief from her symptoms. We both found we had a common interest in healing techniques, and we embarked on a journey of camaraderie, dowsing, diet, saunas, and energy healing.

October 1996
Dear Vicki,

Amber and I are covering some exciting areas in energy healing. From the people I have talked with about twenty-first-century disease (about half a dozen), they all seem to have this problem of not being able to differentiate their feelings from others'. I think it's because the disease affects the energy fields around our bodies. The illness makes our energy fields diffuse and expanded (as opposed to normal people, whose energy is compacted and dense). Because of this, our energies are easily able to mingle with other animals' and humans' energy. The problem is that these energies contain our thoughts and feelings, so when they are mixed with thoughts and feelings of others, we become confused as to what we are really thinking. We become muddle-headed and confused. I'll give you an example, Vicki. Not long ago, I looked after a bird that had a broken wing. Its wing had been reset, and I had it in a warm space in the laundry. Now, that night in bed I felt a wave of blackness and intense depression, where previously I was fine, a sensation of being trapped and suffocated. I felt like I wanted to claw my way out of some invisible space, and then all I could see was blood. I eventually reasoned that these weren't my feelings; they must be the bird's. I went into the laundry, and the bird had almost literally clawed itself to pieces, for there was blood everywhere.

Amber and I theorized then that compressing our energy field close to our bodies makes it difficult to pick up another person's or animal's feelings (energy). How do we do this? you may ask. Well, it's by imagination. Imagine that your energy is being sucked close into the body. Once that has been done a couple of times, it's really easy to do. Doing this is working for us. When we pull our energies close to our bodies, we become clearer-headed, more focused, and able to differentiate more easily our thoughts from those of others.

Another thing that energy-healing does is that it brings to the fore feelings that have been suppressed. I did Amber's energy treatment the other day, and I felt a wave of intense anger from her body.

"Amber, you need to get really angry. Let it go. It's making you sick," I said.

Amber replied, "I know. I've been feeling pissed off. What can I do? Why am I so angry all the time?"

I said, "I don't know, but we're going to find out. Come on. We're going to do a field trip to The Point to find out."

"What, now?" said Amber.

"Yep," I said.

"I, Amber Watson, want to say *fuck!*" Amber screamed as we stood on the rocks at The Point. Why do things have to be so fucking hard?" she screamed as we both hurled large rocks into the water. We watched them make gigantic waves, heard the large thuds as the rocks sank far down into the blue clear waters.

"More, Amber. Come on, there's no one here—we can scream to our hearts' delight."

"Vicki, I feel silly," Amber hissed.

"No, don't worry; it's more important to get rid of the anger." With that I picked a large rock and cracked it onto another.

"Come on, Amber, do it—scream out whatever's in your head."

She screamed, "Fucking hell! Why am I like this? It's not fair!"

Well, Vicki, anyone looking on would have thought we were crazy, but it did help. We both screamed ourselves hoarse over the shittiness of our lives. Afterwards, we sat looking at the river, watching the tugs passing by. Amber said it was the first time that she had let herself experience being angry with the mess she called her life.

"I feel great," she yelled out across the river.

Other things Amber and I have found out have been the commonalities of our illness. We have found out that highs and lows characterize it. That is, we would experience a few weeks of feeling energetic, to the point of mania, as well as very anxious and allergic, followed by a depression and extreme fatigue. We worked out that at least we could try to pace ourselves through the anxiety and avoid things we're allergic to. During the fatigue we should rest in the knowledge it will eventually lift. It's hard, but what is great is that I have someone to discuss this with and to work through the problems I face. I'm not alone in this hell. I've taught Amber how to pendulum, and it works for her too, so we are doing dowsing once a week.

Dear Vicki,

I've been doing quite a few energy healings. Not many on people with allergies, unfortunately. I'd like to explore the commonalities of energy fields in those people. So far I've only worked with a dog with severe allergies, apart from Amber and myself. What I found in common with these energies was a sense of energy that's large, diffuse, and watery in texture. When I release this energy, the individual is less allergic and more relaxed, which is great. This procedure needs to be done every few days or so; before the relief, however, the individual will be in floods of tears and experiencing sadness. This eventually lifts, leaving them feeling much better. I can't talk for the dog, but she is relaxed after her treatments and seems to gain some relief from her allergic symptoms. I don't know how this treatment would work on an anaphylactic reaction (i.e., stop her from experiencing a severe reaction), but I suspect, in the absence of being near immediate medical intervention, a treatment may buy some time before help arrives.

An amazing thing has been happening, the more I do treatments. A voice speaks to me. I don't get the images in my head any more, just this voice that tells me what type of balancing I should be doing, the types of supplements needed and their biochemical status, and what is needed to rectify the problem. This voice is male and doesn't sound like my usual head voice. It is scientific, analytical and, according to my clients, spot on. I've been told it's my spirit guide, but I haven't actively sought one. I don't know how I've even done it. It's a bit spooky. Perhaps I'm schizophrenic! It also happens when I dowse, and it's always right. It's as if dowsing with its yes/no answers is too slow.

November 1996
Dear Vicki,

I'm not making much money out of energy healing, and to be honest, it simply tires me out, because it releases suppressed emotions and because I'm still not well enough to go out and sell myself. For these reasons I've decided on the pension. I don't want to bludge; it's that it's embarrassing and worrying to be on sickness benefits and be assessed every three months by my horrible doctor. I have found a MCS specialist, and I've now applied for the pension.

Vicki, I've found that spirituality alone doesn't pay the bills and that being on the pension will make me eligible for Commonwealth Rehabilitation Services (CRS). I've been so bored with staying at home; my mind wants some action, something that will give me a reason to a get up in the mornings. For this reason I've applied for the CRS.

22

New Directions

Dear Vicki,

The lovely woman at CRS was so helpful. She said she would find me a placement at the theatre company. I've agreed. I may have allergies and fatigue, but what are the things I am able to do?

Dear Vicki,

Today was my first day at the theatre company. I took my mask and cotton gloves just in case I have to read or do photocopying. My rehabilitation officer will assess me every few weeks, and I'm starting at three hours each week and getting paid for it, as well as petrol.

"Hello, my name is Barbara," said this trendy, tall, brunette woman. She took me by the hand and shook it. I instantly warmed to her. "I'm the receptionist and the everything-else-extra-that-needs-doing person," she laughed with smiling brown eyes. I looked around the office; there were three others there; one was a technician, dressed in black, called Tony. I've seen her before. *How cool, working with all that technical equipment, shining lights, doing the sound. I want to do that,"* I thought. The other two were looking officious as they worked on their computer screens.

"This person over here ..." I looked to a crumpled dressed unshaven man, "is the director of the company. Tim."

Oh my God, I want to be a writer-director, I thought as my heart skipped a beat. There were so many things I wanted to do in theatre. This was a dream come true. My eyes shone with enthusiasm. The office was a bit scruffy, but everyone in it looked trendy, and Vicki, the way they spoke to one another showed respect. It certainly wasn't like nursing.

"Today you'll be helping me do the pays on the computer," said Barbara. I was in heaven.

Dear Vicki,

Work isn't easy. I've been having difficulty increasing my hours simply because I'm too tired. Also, the smell from the photocopier comes through my mask and makes me feel terrible. An even worse thing is that I'm sensitive to the electromagnetic radiation of the computer. Whenever I look at the screen I get tired and dyslexic with numbers. I couldn't do the pay because of this. I've asked to try stage management instead. Tony said there's a play on now that needs an assistant stage manager. Who needs reception work, anyway? I have to wear cool black clothing and run around looking important. The show's running for two weeks, and if I do nothing prior to coming to and immediately after the show, I'll be able to do it, I hope.

Dear Vicki,

Today I helped with the sets. I was in heaven.

"Vicki can you stand over here, please? We need to see how the lights are when Anna stands here for this part of the play," said Tim. I stood centre stage, with the warm, dazzling lights shining on my face. I was on fire. I mean, I could sense the audience who would watch this play. To me the air felt electric. Me? Me? I was helping to create this vision. I could smell the wood and sawdust of the new stage. I watched in awe as Tim and Tony created a fairyland of light and ambience. Shadows danced across the stage.

"Vicki, this play relies solely on lighting, acting, and a few props in between the acts. I want you to put out the props as quickly as possible." Then, Vicki, the pièce de résistance—the mixing board—and I'm in love! Everything was timed down to the last second or part thereof. The lighting board coincided with the sound tracks, and eventually I will be given the opportunity to operate the mixing board! It's tricky, but I think I can do it.

Dear Vicki,

Opening night was a buzz. I organized to stay with Mum and Dad so that I could have my meals cooked and I could concentrate on resting for the remainder of my time when I wasn't working. I felt really cool dressed in black, collecting the tickets, running the bar, and preparing the stage. I did some sound and lighting. I've found the cast to be really friendly. We technicians had a special bonfire at midnight down at The Point. The really sad thing is I recognize that I'm not well enough to do this type of work for any length of time. As it was, I had to take several nights off during the show, and a week after, to recuperate, because I was just too exhausted. Oh, Vicki, what am I going to do? I've finished my length of time at Junction, and I couldn't increase my time there to more than a few hours a week. The report from my rehabilitation officer recommends that I'm not well enough to do any work. I'm devastated.

December 1996
Dear Vicki,

Last night and for the past few weeks I've had the same dream. I'm back at Latrobe University. I'm sitting in the cold tomb-like lecture theatre with no windows, taking notes and looking at a projection screen. I can't make out the subject, and I'm squinting to see what's written on the board. I keep thinking, "I finished university nine years ago. What am I doing here?" Yet night after night I'm at university, writing, taking notes, and studying for exams. Then, Vicki, it dawned on me I could go to university and study theatre part-time. I inquired about it, but the course is full time. I was initially disappointed, but then I met a woman whose name was Sue, and she knew someone who was a lecturer in film, and her course was part time. I found out about the course, and Vicki, it's exactly what I want to do. You learn all these cool things, like filming, editing, scriptwriting, making documentaries, and how films are created. What's more, prior recognition for my B.Behav.Sc!

January 1997
Dear Vicki,

It's really like it was in my dream—hundreds of sweaty bodies cramped on plastic seats in an airless room. I'm wearing my mask, feeling self-conscious at being stared at. The mask scratches my face. It feels hot, and my glasses fog slightly.

"Sorry, the air conditioner's on the blink," says the apologetic lecturer. As he speaks I pick up my pen. Am I allergic to the plastic? I wonder. I become aware that the bare skin on the back of my legs is touching plastic. I'm allergic to this type of plastic. I feel queasy; perhaps I made a mistake being here. Suddenly we're plunged into darkness, and a film rolls.

"I want you think about how film is made. It's made up of hundreds of shots. There are varying techniques used to make these shots look as if they flow on together. If you look closely you can see this …" I was sold as I saw the images dance in front of me.

That was my first day. I loved it. In order to get there, I had to plan. That is something my illness has taught me to do: plan, plan, to the nth degree. Initially I contacted the disability officer, who was very helpful to me. She offered to send an introductory letter to my lecturers stating that I needed a perfume-free, non-toxic environment and extra time to complete essays and exams because my illness affected my cognition. I was even offered lessons on Dragon Dictate, which was a computer programme that worked on voice command, thus saving my arms from being tired from typing. I wasn't very good at it and I didn't persevere, but it was good to know that the database was available if my condition deteriorated. I didn't have a computer, but the university has them in the library. Luckily my Dad had one, and I could use his. A friend of mine with CFS was able to use a loan laptop that was available from the disability officer to study at home. Initially I also had problems with the electromagnetic field of the computer. I circumnavigated this problem by wearing filtered glasses, having a computer filter screen, and timing my exposure for, say, ten minutes to the computer and then taking a few moments' break. I also purchased a special medallion that was supposed to deflect electromagnetic radiation. I don't know whether it worked, but after doing all these things, I was gradually able to sit in front of my computer for a couple of hours a day. I also joined the disability group. I only went to a few of their occasions, but each time I went, I was humbled and more determined to succeed at university. These people, one a quadriplegic, others severe schizophrenics, had to fight just to live each day, let alone study.

All in all I directed five short films during my time at university. No mean feat, since to be able to direct was a very much sought-after position, one that was very competitive. Each time we shot a film I'd work twelve-hour days with very few breaks, and by the end,

I'd have to be carried home, unable to talk or walk. It was if I had cerebral palsy; my limbs shook and my words would not come out. Then I'd need a week's solid rest before I could do anything else. Eventually I made it. I only did one or two subjects at a time, and quite often, owing to ill health, I would have extensions. My health was annoying. If I had walked too much, for example, I'd have no power in my legs even for driving. Often I had to tie a belt under my foot and lift it up and down to maintain a certain speed. Other times, if I used the computer too much, the world would be a blur for several days, making it impossible to read. Most of the time I felt I was thinking in cement; my head was so muddled and unclear. I would often forget what I'd read, having to read and reread my study over and over. Eventually I obtained my degree, only to realize that it is a hard, competitive world out there. I found the film industry took up too much of my energy, and I couldn't stand the bitchiness. For this reason, for the time being, I'm not pursuing a film career. I felt I needed a job that was real and dealt with the human condition rather than being a false world based on competition.

Just before 1999, whilst making a documentary, I was hit on the head by a flowerpot, of all things! I developed concussion that went to confusion, in which I couldn't tell the concussion's symptoms from twenty-first century disease. I remember that time vividly, as it was a terrifying experience. I was doing a shoot called *Cadaver Dogs*. It had an exciting premise, dogs that uncover dead bodies for the police. I was so excited that I'd won the pitch to do it and had excellent crew. Prior to filming I had spent days in bed, dizzy with pounding headache and with TV making it worse. I hoped against all hope I could do the shoot. As I thought of this, I would cry all the time, for no apparent reason. I soldiered on—I had to, as I was the director. As the director, I was supposed to be the most important person making the film, since I had to organize and design the look of the film. I ended up directing from bed, with the crew coming to my bedside for instructions. As to looking down the eyepiece of the camera, I nearly passed out with nausea each time I had to arrange a shoot. I ended up in hospital with a mental breakdown. Apart from being a heartache in a difficult life, my breakdown was actually a breakthrough. This was because during my stay in hospital I was able to cope with what used to be, for me, a toxic environment. I had no ill effects from the smells of the carpets, air conditioning, and antiseptics. I think that the drugs I was given which calmed my anxiety and stopped my moods from swinging considerably helped. I can only surmise that they helped because (I think) they stopped me from experiencing a learnt response (anxiety and fear of being allergic) when I came in contact with certain substances, and I began to live without fear of being sick. In other words, I think that there comes a time when the illness has ended but the body, having learnt to respond in dramatic ways, forgets how to act normally. It's as if the body is stuck in high alert all the time, even when the danger is well and truly over.

Since that time I haven't looked back in relation to my allergies. I am on medication for my mental illness, but only low doses, and I might be for life. Who cares, when I feel normal, vibrant, and in control most of the time in my emotions. It's been six years now, and I have had no allergies since then. I don't write a journal any more. I'm now doing part-time work and am studying my graduate diploma in creative writing. I'm working as a registered nurse in an aged-care facility, and I love it. Nursing was something I had to grow into—it's real. I have a life, and I write and make documentaries. I have had a partner now for the past five years; we even made a commitment and are buying a house. There's almost nothing I can't do now, if I put my mind to it.

23

How I Did It

DOWSING

The pendulum taps into the subconscious—the part of us that is all- knowing. To tap into this ability, use a piece of string or chain with a heavy object tied to it. A necklace or tea bag on a string is ideal. Hold the string between the thumb and the first finger, letting it dangle. Imagine that you are talking to an all-knowing part of your self. Let go of the need to control the string. Don't try to influence the string. Ask your all-knowing self to swing the pendulum for a "yes" response. The pendulum, seemingly of its own accord, should then swing in either a clockwise or anticlockwise direction dependent on what your subconscious determines. Then repeat this process for a "no" response. The pendulum should revolve in the opposite direction. Ask for an "I don't know" signal, which would be more imprecise, such as swinging from side to side or not at all. Practise this process until it becomes really easy. Next, ask the subconscious, "Is now a good time to be dowsing?" If it isn't, try again later. It may well be that you are too tired to obtain an accurate reading. If the pendulum answers yes, go ahead and practise. Question it regarding a list of foods that you have been eating, asking the pendulum to give you a yes or a no for food sensitivity. To improve your accuracy and prove to yourself that this works, try this simple game. You need a small ball and three inverted cups. Place the ball under one of the inverted cups and shuffle them around. Next, use the pendulum to determine which cup it is under. It is accurate with practice at least 85 per cent of the time (Macmanaway, 2001).

BODY ORDER DOWSING

By using body order dowsing techniques, combined with regular chiropractic, you can determine where you are in regards to self-healing and which area, whether it be the body, mind, or spirit, needs to be worked on first. Once the area to be worked on is determined, you should then write down a list of every possible thing that might be done to improve that area. Next, dowse this list to find out what is the most salient thing needing attention. To be effective, you should do this every few days during an acute phase of illness and then weekly as your condition improves. First of all, to get a baseline, ask your subconscious what percentage of body order (BO) you are in. Keep a log, and once a week record the improvement or deterioration of your BO. If your BO is improving, there is no need to do any BO dowsing that day. If it is the same as last time or worse, you need to dowse.

To do BO dowsing, write down the following:

M
I
N
D

B
O
D
Y

S
P
I
R
I
T

Then dowse which area needs attention the most. Once this is established, write down all the things you think you might need in that area. These will be based on hunches, research, strong likes or dislikes, and cravings. For example, if I selected *body* as the most salient, I might have a list that looks something like this:

Diet
Exercise
Rest
Massage
Acupuncture

If dowsing revealed that *diet* was the most important thing to improve BO, then you would write down a list of things that you need you improve in this area, that is, a list of food that you have eaten recently, foods that could enhance health (such as shiitake mushrooms), or foods that you need to avoid. You might also ask, "Do I need supplements?"

Once you have done this, ask if there are any other areas that need attention at that time. If the answer is yes, go through the whole process again. Usually you only need to do this process once more, if that. The reason is that once these changes have been made the body is able to start healing itself, and a completely new set of circumstances will be present in a few days' time.

ENERGY TREATMENTS

Energy treatments are good for many things, such as relieving anxiety, physical pain, and the reaction to allergies, as well as releasing emotions and lifting depression. They can be administered in a number of ways.

1. There are seven energy centres (chakras) in the body that are important for the normal, healthy functioning of the body. They are as follows: the crown, brow, throat, heart, solar plexus, the sacral and base of the pelvis which is the sexual region… Dowse over each chakra to determine whether or not it is blocked. Once the blocked zones are established, use the pendulum to work out where to place your hands on your subject for the best healing to take place. Let your imagination and intuition guide you. Picture yourself surrounded by golden light and healing energy coming into your head and passing out through your hands into the person you are healing. Imagine you are safe and protected from harm. You may experience warmth or coolness and the need to move your hands to another part of the body. If that is the case, it is all right to do so. Or you might see symbols in your mind's eye. If you do, try to work out what they mean to you and to the person you are trying to heal. Healing time varies, but it usually takes between half an hour and an hour. You may feel as though you're pulling stuff out of the other person's body. This is the blocked energy. Envisage yourself pulling it out and flicking it away. Imagine that this energy is converted and going towards the good of the planet. Once you feel you have finished, visualize your energy as separate from the other person's. Ask for feedback, and keep a journal of

your treatments. Remember that when you carry out energy treatments on others, you are also treating yourself; emotions trapped in your body and energy field will be released. Drink lots of water, because this sort of work takes up energy, so you need water to replenish yours.

2. Solo energy healing is done the same way as above, except on yourself. If, for example, you are feeling muddle-headed and confused, it could be because your energy field is dispersed and expanded. It makes sense to bring in the energy. One way of doing this is by imagining that your energy field is being held in your hand. In your mind's eye, gently push this energy closer together to form a ball. Hold it, and feel it getting more compact. This will cause your own energy around your body to be drawn more tightly in, and you will feel more clear-headed.

3. A similar method of solo energy healing can also be used for anxiety. Imagine that the energy is your fear. Hold it in your hand and cradle it, be gentle, and stroke it. Now compact it so it forms a hard white pearl. Feel it. This pearl is beautiful, even though it contains all your fears. But they can't escape. Each time you start to feel tense, picture the pearl again, and imagine that all the fear is in there, but this time it can't harm you any more.

4. Alternatively, you may be feeling depressed. Do the above, as described in point 1, but also imagine that the depression is blackness, and this blackness is a cloud. Imagine it lifting outside of your body. Then again, you might imagine the depression as being made of black glass and see yourself smashing it with a hammer until all the depression is gone. Your imagination can be limitless in this healing technique.

5. Pain is also an interesting sensation to ameliorate. Imagine that the pain is being touched gently and held. Picture it being gently drawn out of the body and into the atmosphere. Pull out the threads, the source of the pain, and remind yourself that there is no need to hurt any more.

6. Couples energy treatments can be used when couples can no longer discuss an issue and there seems no way out. Ask the couple to sit facing each other, looking into one another's eyes. Get them to hold hands, and ask them if they are really willing to resolve their issues. If they say they are, continue. Carry out the same procedure as outlined in point 1, and then imagine that the blocks to the couple's communication are lifting. Imagine drawing out the strands of discontent. Ask them to verbalize any words they may feel coming to the fore. Request that they ask out loud for the grace to let go of the things they feel are blocking them from truly communicating. Emotions will arise. Invite the couple to ponder these feelings and not to judge them. Within a relatively short time you will find that both parties are honestly communicating. The blocks will have been removed energetically.

Useful Books
Macmanaway, Dr P. *Dowsing for Health*, Amness Publishing Ltd., 2001
Stein, Diane. *All Women are Healers*, Crossing Press, 1990

DIET

1. I followed no set diet, but the common sensitivities are peanuts, wheat products, dairy, sugar, and nightshades, such as tomatoes and potatoes. This is a good place to start when you make a list of things you eat, in preparation for dowsing. If wheat products come up, helpful alternatives are buckwheat flour (which isn't wheat), rice, corn, soy, and maize. Alternatives for milk products are soy, rice milk, goat's milk, and Nuttelex. Nuttelex is a margarine/butter substitute. Organic food is the best, but once the body has recovered sufficiently, well-washed vegetables will do. There are many special diets that have been suggested by others, such as the Hay Diet or rotation diet, but I've found that they deny me any pleasure. Sometimes it pays to have a little of what one's sensitive to. Dowse to find out how often you can have these foods.

2. Supplements and vitamins are also useful and need to be included when dowsing for body order. The most useful vitamins and supplements to me are these:

Chelated magnesium: for irritability and headaches

Tri-salts: a combination of bicarbonate of soda and other products, available from some chemists. These de-acidify the blood, relieving headaches and confusion.

Tonic water for muscle spasm, taken periodically. It's not recommended to take this all the time, because it is toxic in large doses.

Kali phos (kalium phosphoricum): a homeopathic medicine for muscle spasm

Slippery elm: used for abdominal cramps and wind pain

Echinacea: for colds and minor infections

Shitake mushrooms: to boost the immune system

Vitamin C: one gram taken twice daily to build up the immune system

Multivitamin and mineral supplements, including B12 injections, to boost energy

Saunas: at least twice a week, to sweat out the toxins

Avoid antibiotics. They'll make you very sick. Instead, use natural alternatives as much as possible.

A useful book on special diets is *Toxic Chemical-Free Living,* by Trixie Whitmore.

CREATING AN ENVIRONMENTALLY FRIENDLY HOUSE IN THE CITY

The house in its entirety should be newish but not too new. That is, it should not have been recently painted, carpeted, or refurbished. On the other hand, it shouldn't be too old, meaning containing dust, mould, or mildew. It should have wooden floors and use electricity rather than gas. It should be freestanding and away from neighbours who are renovating or who use pesticides. It should be away from main roads and traffic. If it is not, then seriously consider moving to somewhere that fits most of these criteria. Before putting anything new in the house, dowse the item. Sometimes all it takes is a couple of months for the new smell to disappear or a wash to make the item suitable for the house. Ensure that visitors have been notified that they must not wear perfumed soap, hairsprays, perfumes, or deodorant. When cleaning the house, use all-natural products, and wear a gas mask and cotton gloves for handling house dust. Pets may also be problem. If you are very attached yet sensitive to them, vacuum every day. Wear a mask when close to them and cotton gloves for patting them—they don't care what you look like.

CLEANING AGENTS FOR THE BATHROOM

Bicarbonate of soda mixed with lemon on a sponge for the basin

A teaspoon of vinegar mixed with hot water for the toilet bowl and cleaning the floors

Newspaper and hot water for the mirrors and windows

Wash yourself with Sorbolene lotion, no soap, and use only water for hair-washing at your most allergic times. Dowse to see if you can tolerate a little soap. Some people are allergic to the water itself. You can purchase a special shower nozzle that takes out the chemicals.

WASHING CLOTHES/FABRICS/DISHES

Try to wear all-natural products, such as cotton and wool. Avoid man-made fibres, because you may be allergic. Don't wear clothing that is new; wash clothes at least two or three times before wearing. If you must use soap, use a perfume-free soap powder, such as Black and Gold, because this reduces the risk of sensitivities. Wash your clothes with soap every alternative wash. This cuts down the contact with soap. Velvet dishwashing soap, in a wire basket, is ideal for washing dishes.

THE BEDROOM

Vacuum the mattress weekly with a good vacuum cleaner. Have the mattress off the floor. Use cotton or flannelette sheets and all-natural fibres for rugs. Damp-dust daily. Don't buy new rubber or foam for the mattress. Rubber, whether old or new, is especially bad, and should be avoided at all costs. For this reason, avoid rubber-backed curtains. Use louvres or blinds to block out light and heat.

PESTS

Keep spaces clear and clean. Avoid using pesticides. A fly swat is the ideal alternative or a mozzie zapper. Citronella oils or candles can also be beneficial, but I found I was allergic to them as well, so I couldn't use them.

PERSONAL PRODUCTS

Deodorants such as crystal rocks can be used. Tampons should be organic cotton. The others contain bleaches and traces of pesticides, so they can make you very sick. Alternatively, use sea sponges or towel pads.

Useful books: *Toxic Chemical-Free Living*, by Trixie Whitmore

SMUDGING AND CREATING A SACRED SPACE/MEDICINE WHEEL

Smudging is used to purify self and spaces—in other words, it gets rid of negative energy. Smudging is similar to dressing, especially for the spirit world. Special herbs, such as rosemary, lavender, sage, or eucalyptus, are dried out and bundled together. The bundles are called smudge sticks. They are burnt and the smoke wafted in the air and over the body. Native Americans gather the leaves used for this process by asking out loud for the plants' permission. They are usually collected at full moon. Ceramic bowls are used to contain the herbs. The individual sits and wafts the smoke over the head, the body, and then the feet; it's like washing with smoke.

To create a sacred space/medicine wheel, place objects (such as stones) in a circle, with the four directions of north, south, east, and west. These are representative of fire, earth, air, and water, respectively. Circle the space with a lit smudge stick. Smudge yourself before entering the circle. Ask permission of the East, which represents air and logic, to enter the wheel. Next move to the fire (North) position; this is passion. Call forth these qualities with your hands outstretched, really concentrating on them. Following that, move to the West position;—this is the direction of emotions and flowing water—and concentrate on these qualities. After this, move to the South position. This is the growth and grounded portion of the wheel. Next move to the centre of the circle and think of Mother Earth. Hold up your hands and think of the sky/spirit/Father Sky. Once this is done, you have created a sacred space, one where you can reflect and feel at peace and free from negativity. You may leave this space permanently set up by exiting the circle by the west door, giving thanks as you pass through it. Alternatively, you may wish to close the circle. This is done by saying farewell to the six positions, from the sky to the earth, to the south, east, north, and leaving by the western door.

Books: *Buffalo Woman Comes Singing,* by Brooke Medicine Eagle, Ballantine Books, New York, 1991

APPLYING FOR DISABILITY SUPPORT PENSION AND THE ADVANTAGES

First of all, gain a specialist in CFS/MCS to get the diagnosis confirmed. To find these specialists, ring up the CFS/MCS Society in your nearest city. Ask to apply for the Disability Support Pension if you have severe CFS/MCS. Acquire the forms from Centre Link, fill them out, and lodge them along with your specialist's diagnosis and prognosis. Don't be talked out of going on the pension if you feel you need it. If you go on the pension, you can utilize it to make your recovery. Once Centre Link has your forms, they will ask you to be assessed by the state medical doctor. Be honest with these doctors, as they like people who want to use the pension to help themselves recover. The assessment process takes a month or so.

Once accepted for disability pension (beside the usual subscription and travel discounts) you are eligible for the following:

1. Commonwealth Rehabilitation Services (CRS), whereby the government will place you in employment, pay for training if it's not too dear, and give emotional support whilst doing it.

2. Pensioner Supplement Loan, whereby you are given approximately $60 a fortnight to aid with studying. You are eligible for this on top of the pension if you are studying at least a quarter of the normal study workload. Alternatively, if you're really strapped for cash, you can trade in the $60 to gain a $120 loan per fortnight that is only paid back (with interest) when you are earning a sizeable income. If you never earn that much, you never have to pay it back!

3. Emergency housing or a trust home. You are more eligible for these if you get the written back-up from friends, the doctor, and other health professionals. The South Australian Housing Trust will pay for a one-way furniture moving, but only if you ask.

STUDYING AT UNIVERSITY

You are eligible to seek assistance from the disability officer, who will introduce you to others and to your lecturers. He or she will provide you with aids, such as a laptop, or give you access to the hands-free Dragon Dictate voice-activated writing programme. The officer will also help you gain access to counselling and assignment extensions. Sit down and write a list of your special requirements. You may need a scooter to ride on or a disability-parking sticker.

PHOTOCOPYING

Avoid this as much as possible. The library has facilities to do this for you, provided you give them sufficient warning. If you don't have this facility, barter with someone else to do it for you. Failing that, as a last resort wear your mask for the fumes and cotton gloves to protect your hands from the lead.

COMPUTING

Limit your time at the computer. Time it for, say, ten minutes, and then take a minute's break, gradually increasing the time. The new flat-screen computers put out less electromagnetic radiation, so use one of these if possible. Wear glasses that screen ultraviolet glare. You may also like to try special electromagnetic deflection machines, but these are very expensive, and I don't know whether they work anyway.

24

The Present and Bipolar Disorder

ife hummed along pretty well in 2007. I had a loving partner of six years and had bought a house and a Toyota RAV4. These were things I'd previously only dreamt of having! I was living the dream, with enough money to be comfortable and the ability to concentrate on making friends and studying. It was during this time that I attended Tabor College and studied creative writing. Whilst there, I became interested in Christianity and became a Christian. Unfortunately, peace did not reign for long, because in 2013 I had another breakdown, just when I had been feeling safe and secure. Out of the blue came a reaction to some herbal medication I was taking. This, in turn, sent me off on a psychotic episode, an experience during which I thought a woman at work was an alien and that I had mothered an alien child.

Even as I write this, I cringe. When will these notions of aliens leave me? I remember thinking that the woman from work could connect with me telepathically and we could spend hours conversing this way. Of course, in reality, none of this was true. One good thing came out of my experience: I was able to forgive the so-called aliens from abducting me all those years ago. I did this by reasoning that the aliens were like conservationists who captured, branded, and returned people to the world and that they had no idea of the negative impact they had on our species but were doing it to help save humanity. It was from this perspective that I learnt to forgive them and finally put them to rest.

During this time I had a newish GP, one who didn't think I had had Chronic Fatigue or MCS in the past. She believed I had a mental disorder and referred me to a psychiatrist who diagnosed me as bipolar type 1. This is characterized by episodes of extreme highs followed by deep depression, with periods of psychosis. It turns out bipolar people are also very sensitive to odours and suffer from extreme fatigue. Once again, the baby had been thrown out with the bath water. Have all my visions and my experiences been due to unstable memories? Was even my initial alien experience a psychosis? What can I trust to be the truth? I like to think something untoward happened, and I snapped three times; in fact, to the point that it led me to the diagnosis of bipolar type 1.

It was a painful time for me. I was placed on lithium, a mood stabilizer; Faverin, an antidepressant; and amilsulpride, an antipsychotic. My mood swings stopped, and my allergies went away. Apparently, bipolar people suffer a lot from allergies and sensitivities if not medicated.

Where does it leave me now, given my life experiences? I don't know exactly, but I can say that going on the tablets has stopped the highs, the nightmares, and the hallucinations—whilst simultaneously dulling down my personality, which I'm not too keen on. It's easy to say my mind over the years has played tricks, but I still want to honour my original experience as something out of the ordinary happening, which culminated in bipolar disorder years later. I also believe dowsing helped me live with my sensitivities. By the time I met the current doctor, my allergic nature was almost gone.

As for my relationship with God, just when I thought I had him buttonholed, a whole new universe has opened up. The Old Testament paints God as a harsh taskmaster and warlord. As you can guess, I don't relate to that God. Yet in the New Testament, Jesus is loving, forgiving, and active for peace—principles by which I live my life. I'm currently attending a progressive church, but given my experience I want to believe in miracles and the presence of the Holy Spirit in the everyday. My experiences have opened the door to the miraculous. I take some of this into my day job, working with the disabled.

There are five possible conclusions that can be drawn regarding the mission. The first one is that, since I am bipolar, my experience was a psychotic episode. Even if this were true, it shows the deep-seated yearning to know God that has preoccupied me these last thirty years. So it had value. Value aside, it doesn't account for the three other people involved in the mission, unless one considers group psychosis, which is unlikely, since Kerry and Carla weren't acquainted with me before the incident. It also doesn't explain how the car drove by itself. Nor can this conclusion explain the hypnotherapy sessions in which I stated I'd been abducted by aliens and that I had been in contact with them as a child.

The second conclusion is that it was God calling us. As I had a view of God as a harsh taskmaster, someone to be feared, God may have appeared to me as such, because that is what I understood God to be. If one accepts this premise, it doesn't explain the presence of aliens, however. Perhaps they were working alongside God to save our planet and in fact we were on a mission to save it. This would explain the car driving by itself, the books in Barr Smith library, and Aggie and Hector and the devil trying to stop me.

That the devil tricked me is the third possible conclusion. The devil persuaded me to commit to a mission. His aim was to confound me and do harm by playing on my sense of justice. I've certainly had my share of illness and madness attributed to the mission. But why was the devil lurking round, trying to seduce me, when he already had me, if it were him responsible for the mission? Why, then, if the devil wished us harm, did he organize/orchestrate an accident at which a tow truck was on the standby? Why did he lead us to people to confide in?

The fourth conclusion is that there were only aliens involved. They orchestrated the accident. They found suitable sensitive people and convinced us to go on a mission. We were, in fact, on a mission to save the planet.

The fifth conclusion is that God does speak to us, as does our intuition. Church has shown me that God does talk to us. However, one needs a discerning ear to determine whether or not it is God. Hence, dowsing is used to bleed out the static, so that one can pick up the pure message.

Epilogue

At the end of 2007, as I look back over my life, I've see that I've had the worst but also some of the best of times. MCS/CFS is certainly one of the most terrifying diseases. I cannot emphasize that enough, because with this disease there is no safe place. My body was in a state of war; it was fighting against the twenty-first century's pollutants. Each moment of that time was like being in hell. I had to literally drag my body along. At times I was so weak that I had to remain in one spot as if transfixed. Then, when I had the energy or was hauled by others, I would go to bed to sleep, seemingly for weeks, until I had enough energy to get up. The fear factor was enormous. Whenever I came into contact with an allergen, I would taste it constantly in my mouth. I would suddenly, overwhelmingly, feel like committing suicide in a violent, dramatic manner. Spiders, cockroaches, and ants would fill my mind's eye; my stomach would swell up, and I would feel nauseous. I think that I've done my penance in this lifetime!

Many doctors do not accept that the condition exists, yet if the miners in the old days had ignored the deaths of their caged canaries, they would surely have died. We are those canaries. MCS sufferers indicate that our planet is becoming too toxic, and something must be done before it is too late. Nowadays I buy mostly natural products. I am aware that perfumes and scents can give off toxic odours to others, so I am vigilant in what I wear or use around others. Nevertheless, I am delighted that I am no longer sensitive to chemicals.

Recently I had to go into hospital for an MRSA wound infection. I had to go on intravenous antibiotics, and even that way, I tolerated them with no problems at all. I think illness is a very personal thing, and the recovery from illness is specific to the individual. I believe that dowsing allowed me to determine what I needed in order to heal. From the research I have done on dying clients, I have found that those who recover or go into remission do so because they discovered what their bodies specifically needed to heal. There is no formula, such as diet, meditation, and so on, but rather a combination of factors that contain spiritual, mental, and physical elements. If I could have popped a pill for this illness, I would certainly have done so, but that was not to be the case. I have learnt and experienced so much. This illness honed my intuition and strengthened my bond with God—an entity I would not have made it without through my miraculous recovery.

www.ingramcontent.com/pod-product-compliance
Lightning Source LLC
Chambersburg PA
CBHW032055020426
42335CB00011B/355